Strategic Allocation and Management of
CAPITAL IN HEALTHCARE

T0192952

Strategic Allocation and Management of CAPITAL IN HEALTHCARE

A GUIDE TO DECISION MAKING

Second Edition
Jason H. Sussman

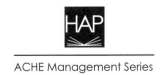

ACHE Management Series

Library of Congress Cataloging-in-Publication Data

Names: Sussman, Jason H., author.
Title: Strategic allocation and management of capital in healthcare : a guide
   to decision making / Jason H. Sussman.
Other titles: Healthcare executive's guide to allocating capital
Description: Chicago, IL : HAP, [2018] | Series: ACHE management series |
   Revision of: Healthcare executive's guide to allocating capital. c2007. |
   Includes bibliographical references.
Identifiers: LCCN 2017015564| ISBN 9781567939149 (alk. paper) | ISBN
   9781567939163 (xml) | ISBN 9781567939170 (epub) | ISBN 9781567939187 (mobi)
Subjects: LCSH: Medical care—Finance. | Capital.
Classification: LCC RA410.5 .S87 2018 | DDC 615.9—dc23 LC record available at https://lccn
   .loc.gov/2017015564

The paper used in this publication meets the minimum requirements of American National Standard for Information Sciences—Permanence of Paper for Printed Library Materials, ANSI Z39.48-1984. ∞ ™

Acquisitions editor: Janet Davis; Project manager: Andrew Baumann; Cover designers: James Kattinge and Brad Norr; Layout: PerfecType

Health Administration Press
A division of the Foundation of the American
   College of Healthcare Executives
One North Franklin Street, Suite 1700
Chicago, IL 60606-3529
(312) 424-2800

Contents

Foreword

ALLOCATING CAPITAL IS difficult because it involves a series of problems. To quote M. Scott Peck, MD, the author of *The Road Less Traveled* (New York: Simon & Schuster, 2002): "Discipline is the basic set of tools we require to solve life's problems. Without discipline we can solve nothing. With only some discipline we can solve only some problems. With total discipline we can solve all problems."

A number of years ago, I was faced with a significant dilemma as a newly hired chief financial officer for a multistate, $4.5 billion health system. Having received a rating downgrade, and harboring doubts about the best way to move forward as a system, the organization realized that capital allocation was a critical component to our future success. But where to start?

Fortunately, I had the opportunity to be introduced to Kaufman Hall, and specifically Jason Sussman. Jason had been helping other clients with the problem of allocating capital. What emerged for me during the period we worked together was the ultimate capital "Aha!" moment—a true picture of the capital management cycle he described and, more important, the right set of disciplines to execute it well.

After a few years of painstakingly putting in place all the disciplines of a robust capital management cycle, including the capital allocation centerpiece of the process, our organization started making better capital decisions, and results consistently improved. Ultimately, our strong credit rating was restored. In this book, Jason presents the right set of disciplines in a thoughtful, well-organized manner. To executives looking for a quick fix, this probably is not the guide for you, as it requires a commitment to a continuous loop of planning, assessment, analytics, decision making, execution, and reassessment. To executives who are committed to improving their organizations' capital allocation processes through disciplined thought and actions, however, you cannot find a better road map.

My experiences with Jason have been very positive. Together, we have created great value in two large and complex healthcare organizations. His experience, evident throughout this book, has been gleaned from many years of working with healthcare providers across the country. I have heard so many positive, reinforcing comments about his work that I am confident you will find this book enormously helpful in moving your organization forward in a time of great challenges, yet also of great opportunity.

Peter L. DeAngelis Jr.
Executive Vice President, Chief Financial Officer,
and Chief Administrative Officer
Thomas Jefferson University and Jefferson Health

Preface

When I wrote *The Healthcare Executive's Guide to Allocating Capital* (the first edition of this book) in 2007, my goal was to create a single source of the most successful capital allocation practices for healthcare leaders. It was a time of relative stability during which many organizations were focused on ways to improve management performance and decision making. Given the capital intensity of US healthcare delivery, a disciplined approach to capital allocation and management was one way to make such improvements. Decisions could generate both immediate and longer-term strategic and financial benefits.

As I write this preface to the second edition ten years later, the healthcare environment is anything but stable. Driven by market pressures and accelerated by the Affordable Care Act, healthcare has experienced eight years of steady progress toward payment for value, but the future of payment reform is now unclear. Still, creating value—defined as high-quality care with better patient experience and care outcomes at lower cost—remains a major goal for healthcare. Uncertainty about future payment levels and structures makes the task of identifying the best value-enhancing investments much more difficult. Accordingly, the stakes associated with an organization's ability to allocate and manage capital are higher than ever.

The challenge in preparing this edition was to provide healthcare leaders with even more guidance on this vital decision-making and management process. Discussions with senior management teams and boards made it clear that the fundamentals—which remain as valid today as they were ten years ago—needed to be reinforced and that important issues in the current era needed to be covered as well. This second edition therefore provides full guidance on the corporate finance–based discipline of capital allocation and management and describes its application in the present-day environment.

Although every organization is unique, working with a wide variety of organizations has enabled me to identify common areas of concern and struggle for all organizations on the path to generating real value. No matter how large, complex, or mission driven it is, an organization's ultimate success continues to be a direct function of its ability to manage capital effectively within a consistent and transparent structure that clearly defines accountability. However, to be successful, process design and operation must always reflect changes in the strategic investment focus of organizations responding to dynamic industry. Therefore, updated and new materials in this edition are focused on real organizations and the ways they have successfully addressed areas of common concern in today's evolving healthcare reality. These insights provide a clear sight line into continuing best practices.

Among the issues that organizations of all types must address is the need to appropriately expand the capital allocation and management discipline and tool set to include potential investments that have little or no true capital footprint. By that, I am referring to potential initiatives that include limited, if any, investment in depreciable assets. Investments in population health initiatives and unique physician affiliation arrangements such as clinically integrated networks are two examples. In the not-so-distant past, these types of investments were infrequent and, in many cases, immaterial. Review and approval often flowed through the operating budget process or simply flew under the radar. In today's environment of value creation, however, healthcare organizations are allocating an increasing proportion of their available cash flow to support noncapital initiatives. As a result, the capital allocation and management process needs to adjust to appropriately incorporate these types of initiatives as full-fledged uses of cash flow available for capital investment. Guidance on how to reshape the process is provided throughout this book.

In the ten years since publication of *The Healthcare Executive's Guide to Allocating Capital*, healthcare management practices have changed considerably, increasingly mirroring those of corporate America. Many healthcare organizations are now headed by leaders who embrace the need for analytically based decision making with heightened levels of transparency and accountability. Others are in the process of incorporating such a structure into their organizations. This book is intended to benefit all such organizations, as well as those that have not yet begun the journey.

A book such as this is never the work of one individual. I have certainly benefited from the efforts of my colleagues at Kaufman Hall and from the imagination and focus of the client healthcare organizations with which I have had the privilege to work. New ideas, practical applications, and evolving best practices come from a wide range of sources. Included in this book are the "best of the best" from clients, colleagues, and leading organizations outside of healthcare. These have added a dimension of on-the-ground reality for additional benefit to healthcare leaders.

I want to specifically thank Pete DeAngelis of Thomas Jefferson University for adding his warm and perceptive comments in the book's foreword. Pete and I have worked together toward the common goal of improving organizational decision making for many years. In the course of that journey, we have developed and employed many of the approaches described in this book.

I also sincerely thank Michael Olson from Avera Health, Mary Beth Briscoe from the University of Alabama at Birmingham Health System, and Jimmy Hatcher of Emory Healthcare for providing the descriptions of their organizations' experiences as a means to teach others, as well as for their personal friendship and support.

My colleague Dan Majka, a managing director of Kaufman Hall, deserves special thanks for his chapter-end commentaries that focus on implementation and management issues that make capital allocation and management successful. Dan works closely with senior decision makers in process design and implementation as well as with manager-level planning and implementation teams. Jess Block, a vice president in Kaufman Hall's software practice, helped us select and develop graphics to best illustrate the best-practice functioning of capital allocation and management tools.

I cannot begin to thank Nancy Gorham Haiman enough for her singular efforts as my consultant and the editor for this book. Nancy is a hidden jewel at Kaufman Hall whose experience and ability to coalesce disparate concepts within one book is unmatched. This book and its application throughout the industry will be a testament to Nancy's professional capabilities. I am honored and privileged to have the opportunity to work with Nancy and to call her a friend.

Finally, I want to thank my wife, Karen, without whose support none of this could have happened. Even with all the changes in our lives over these past ten years, Karen has been a constant source of love and support as I traveled the country to work with clients and invested time at home working on this book and other projects. Karen is the glue that holds it all together. I am blessed to have her in my life.

Introduction

WHY THIS BOOK?

Since the publication of the first edition of this book in 2007, the business model used in healthcare for more than a half century has started a profound transformation. Unsustainable national healthcare costs are driving legislation, regulation, and competitive market responses that are rapidly changing healthcare from a volume-based delivery and payment system focused on illness to a value-based system focused on managing population health.

This transformation is placing unprecedented demands on the nation's hospitals, health systems, and related provider organizations. More than at any time in the past, an organization's long-term success and sustainability hinge on smart, strategic investment decisions being made today and in the time since the business model transformation began. Tightening margins increasingly conflict with an ever-expanding list of high-dollar capital needs related to positioning organizations for success under the new model.

Few healthcare organizations have sufficient capital capacity to meet their comprehensive strategic requirements. Their leaders must make choices. How much capital to spend and on which projects or investments are critical decisions with long-term strategic and financial implications.

Executives in the nation's hospitals, health systems, and other provider organizations frequently struggle with making these decisions. As a result, wide variations exist in the decision-making processes used to allocate scarce capital resources. Many organizations implement portions of the best-practice capital allocation and management process described in this book, and they are very adept at managing those aspects. Few organizations, however, address capital allocation and management comprehensively, likely because of the cultural and organizational challenges associated with developing and implementing a strategic capital decision-making process.

Decision-making authority is often a key issue. At what level should capital decisions be made, and who should be involved in their review and approval? Issues surrounding appropriate decision criteria also are critical. Are criteria defined and consistently applied organization-wide? Technical challenges—such as calculation of capital availability, the qualitative and quantitative metrics required for project analysis and review, and the mechanics of integrating the capital allocation and management process with the organization's strategic and financial planning—are numerous and can present significant roadblocks.

Capital management as an integral component of an organization's comprehensive decision-making process is vital to the organization's ability to optimize both its strategic and its financial position. A fully integrated capital allocation and management process provides complete support for the organization's strategic objectives and its ability to sustain successful performance.

GOALS OF THIS BOOK

An organization's ability to address these issues largely determines its strategic future. The design and implementation of a capital decision-making process in healthcare organizations that embraces a corporate finance–like approach is strongly recommended. America's highest-performing organizations in healthcare and other industries use corporate finance principles to manage the strategic and financial risk of their organizations.

Strategic Allocation and Management of Capital in Healthcare: A Guide to Decision Making provides leadership teams with detailed guidance on making the best strategic investments. Like the first edition, it offers a corporate finance–based framework and approach to disciplined capital decision making and management.

In addition, this revised edition reflects the need for the capital decision-making approach to evolve to meet the new environment. It includes examples of the application of concepts using the experiences of specific hospitals and health systems. Developed through engagements and interviews with senior leaders, this material focuses on strategies used to address the barriers these organizations encountered, thereby helping readers to apply the approach in their own organizations. The new edition also includes on-the-ground guidance for managers responsible for the implementation of each chapter's concepts.

Applicable to all healthcare organizations—from small community hospitals to large healthcare systems and physician organizations—*Strategic Allocation and Management of Capital in Healthcare: A Guide to Decision Making* aims to help healthcare organizations achieve and sustain competitive, strategic financial performance.

CONTENTS OVERVIEW

The nine chapters of *Strategic Allocation and Management of Capital in Healthcare: A Guide to Decision Making* outline a best-practice capital management framework and process. Each chapter covers a distinct topic. Examples of framework and process applications in different settings—such as a community hospital and a small, multihospital health system—are provided, as appropriate. Also included is practical guidance for managers who are responsible for implementing the chapter's concepts.

Chapter 1, "Capital Allocation and Management Essentials," defines capital allocation and management and describes how the process is integrally linked through the capital management cycle with the organization's strategic, financial, and capital planning and budgeting processes. The chapter offers a contemporary definition of capital and identifies the types of investments covered through a corporate finance–based approach. It describes the significance of high-quality capital management, outlines common and emergent approaches to allocating capital in healthcare organizations, and concludes with the characteristics of a recommended process.

Chapter 2, "Establishing the Framework," provides guidance on constructing a framework that supports best-practice capital allocation and management. The framework has concrete objectives—consistency, standardization, transparency, known timing, and use of analytics—and it follows core principles, such as equal access to dollars, one-batch review, and portfolio decision making. The chapter also describes how organizations can design or redesign their existing processes and establish a successful governance structure and process calendar that will drive integrated planning and decision making organization-wide.

Chapter 3, "Determining the Capital Constraint," describes the approach executives can employ to quantify the level of capital their organization can afford to invest in the near term and long term. The chapter details the mechanics involved in calculating the capital constraint (net cash available for capital investment), which include determining cash flow, debt proceeds, philanthropic funds, working capital, principal payments, carryforward capital, cash reserve requirements, and other sources and uses of cash. The chapter concludes by explaining why the capital constraint must be defended from common challenges such as those posed by equipment leases; broadened information technology; and new-era calls on capital, such as risk reserves, partnerships, and physician practice acquisitions.

Chapter 4, "Defining the Capital Pools," describes how executives should determine the pools into which the total capital dollars available for investment will be divided. The chapter recommends an approach using three pools: (1) threshold capital, defined as the pool for any capital expenditure above a certain dollar amount that requires comprehensive analysis and centralized review; (2) nonthreshold capital, defined as the pool for requests with associated costs below the threshold dollar amount; and (3) contingency capital, defined as the pool that supports and provides reserves for projects occurring through the other two pools. In addition, the chapter outlines methods for funding and managing the pools.

Chapter 5, "Allocating and Evaluating Nonthreshold Capital," provides a recommended approach to allocating nonthreshold capital, which is typically managed on a decentralized basis, for requests with costs below the threshold dollar amount. The chapter explains how to handle allocation to revenue-generating units as well as to nonprofitable, non-revenue-producing, and small operating units. It also provides information on evaluating nonthreshold capital projects using standardized capital request templates supported by a flexible software tool, an approach that enhances an organization's ability to review the appropriateness of estimated costs and timing and to explore opportunities to combine requests to gain purchasing power and efficiency. A sample template is provided.

Chapter 6, "Evaluating Threshold Capital Investment Opportunities," describes the benefits of using a formal, one-batch process with consistent evaluative criteria to review requests for and allocate capital to large-dollar, threshold capital initiatives. The chapter outlines the key elements of the business plan or standardized project review form that should accompany each request. Corporate finance–based techniques for quantitative return-on-investment analysis are described in detail, including net-present-value analysis and expected-net-present-value analysis. The chapter explains how to quantify qualitative measures and appropriately weight both quantitative and qualitative criteria. Of particular note is the discussion on how to handle large, multiyear projects in an annual process.

Chapter 7, "Selecting Threshold Capital Projects Using a Portfolio Approach," describes how organizations can combine the information obtained through quantitative and qualitative analyses to select a portfolio of threshold projects that balances margin and mission. The chapter outlines the processes involved in constructing both quantitatively based and qualitatively based rankings of projects and in uniting these rankings to select a portfolio of initiatives that will ensure the organization's continued competitive performance.

Chapter 8, "Managing the Postallocation Process," describes what should occur after allocation decisions are made. Activities covered in the chapter include funding review and revalidation, which ensures the integration of new data or information obtained after project approval; decision making regarding the timing of capital spending; handling of any budget deficits or surpluses; addressing emergency and off-cycle requests; ongoing monitoring of project performance; and taking appropriate actions based on performance results.

Chapter 9, "Making It Happen and Keeping It Going," describes the prerequisites for the successful implementation of a high-quality capital allocation and management process. These requirements include education, use of high-quality tools, communication and transparency, and a disciplined implementation plan with a realistic time frame.

CHAPTER 1

Capital Allocation and Management Essentials

THIS CHAPTER IDENTIFIES types of capital resources covered by the capital allocation and management process, defines that process, and describes its significance. The chapter provides details on the decision-making flow or cycle for capital allocation and management, and it outlines the traditional and best-practice approaches to developing and managing the process.

THE NEW DEFINITION OF CAPITAL

A corporate finance approach to capital allocation and management is based on a contemporary, evolving definition of *capital*. This definition extends beyond traditional capital items, such as property, plant, and equipment, to embrace virtually all calls on an organization's cash flow. Essentially everything that might appear on the cash flow statement, including such items as working capital for investment start-ups, joint venture and physician practice investments, health plan investments and reserves required under risk-bearing arrangements, and all other items that take cash out of the organization, should be considered capital uses.

The traditional definition of capital, which focuses only on depreciable assets, is far too narrow to support truly strategic capital management. A broad definition of capital must be accepted as part of the basic structure of the capital allocation and management process because of the breadth of sources for capital deployed through the process and the variety of related capital uses. Exhibit 1.1 provides a comprehensive list of the capital investments that should be subject to the formal allocation and management process. The identified range of investments could as easily apply to a typical community hospital as to a multihospital health system or academic medical center.

Exhibit 1.1 Investments Covered by the Capital Allocation and Management Process

- Facilities, property, and equipment, including information technology
- Business acquisitions and partnerships
- Divestitures and asset monetization
- Equity investments
- Network development
- Managed care investments
- New operating entities, programs, and services
- Program start-up subsidies or expansion
- Physician integration, recruitment, practice purchase, partnership, and other arrangements
- Organization-level (or system) initiatives
- Nontraditional investments, such as post-acute care services

Source: Kaufman, Hall & Associates, LLC. Used with permission.

Applying this broadened definition of capital investments that should be subject to the allocation and capital management process is critical as organizations focus strategic investment away from capacity and toward efficiency and appropriate levels of care. In addition, as discussed in chapter 3, the definition of capital must hold true regardless of the anticipated source of funding for that investment (including leases and philanthropy).

In not-for-profit organizations, capital resources apportioned through the comprehensive capital allocation and management process come from three sources: cash flow from operations, philanthropy, and external debt. Chapter 3 describes these resources in detail.

CAPITAL ALLOCATION AND MANAGEMENT DEFINED

Capital allocation is the strategic process organizations use to make capital investment decisions. Through this process, healthcare executives determine how much capital will be spent and where the organization's scarce capital resources, including cash and debt capacity, will be deployed.

A best-practice *capital allocation and management* process ensures that the organization spends the optimal amount of capital—not too much and not too little.

It also ensures that investment is made in a portfolio of initiatives that provides a positive contribution to the organization's strategic and financial positions.

The capital allocation and management process is not capital budgeting. Exhibit 1.2 describes how the capital budgeting process differs in content and context from the capital allocation and management process.

In contrast to capital budgeting, the capital allocation and management process is comprehensive, with a broad purview over all calls on an organization's cash (listed in exhibit 1.1). The success of the capital allocation and management process is directly tied to the organization's strategic and financial performance. Available dollars are identified on the basis of the organization's long-term strategic and financial vision. Approved allocations of capital are expected to create an overall portfolio that will generate an optimal return over a multiyear period.

Capital allocation and management comprehensively considers the short-term and long-term implications of each potential investment within an overall portfolio of investments. Its focus often extends over three to five years and even beyond—in the case of facility development or the development of new programs, services, or affiliations, for example. The detailed analysis (i.e., business plan) supporting each capital investment proposal provides transparency that enables executives to identify and track key accountabilities, opportunities, risks, and alternative outcomes. A well-devised business plan anticipates potential problems related to individual project or portfolio performance. Problems that do occur can be corrected as they arise, or, in the worst case, exit strategies previously defined in the business plan can be implemented before strategic and financial performance is materially and negatively affected.

Exhibit 1.2 How Capital Budgeting Differs from Capital Allocation

Capital budgeting is the administrative process organizations use to identify and spend "routine" capital that has been allocated. It represents a small piece of the comprehensive capital allocation and management process, typically relating only to minor expenditures that fall under department managers' purview. Larger, more complex capital projects (often designated as "strategic") tend to be reviewed and approved outside the standard capital budgeting process in a planning process managed by a separate set of management players. Capital budgeting has a one-year focus. It is an administratively driven process whose success is measured by such criteria as "time required for completion" and "variance of expenses from budget."

Source: Kaufman, Hall & Associates, LLC. Used with permission.

THE SIGNIFICANCE OF CAPITAL ALLOCATION AND MANAGEMENT

The most important financial decisions made each year by an organization's senior management and ratified by its board relate to how much capital to invest and on which projects and initiatives those dollars will be spent. The long-term success of a healthcare organization depends on the capital investment decisions it makes today. Every decision either increases or decreases organizational value. Investments that protect or improve the organization's net cash flow stream by supporting successful strategies must be part of the long-term strategic and financial plan.

Organizations cannot shrink their way to success. Leadership must act on the knowledge that investments to create ongoing growth are the foundation for the organization's future. Decisions to invest capital must increase organizational value—the organization's ability to generate capital for future investment in known or yet-to-be-defined strategies, maintain or improve its creditworthiness, and accomplish its mission. For every investment that does not generate value (e.g., mission- or community-directed projects), the organization must seek other ways to create equivalent cash flow and value to develop a balanced portfolio. The cumulative effect of incremental decisions determines the organization's overall success. Exhibit 1.3 describes the new view of requirements to achieve growth and scale under healthcare's transforming business model.

High-performing organizations place a high priority on the formal allocation of capital because they understand that existing capital capacity, defined as the amount of debt- and cash flow–based capital an organization can generate and support, is a function of past performance. The creation and regeneration of capital capacity depend on the organization's continuing ability to make value-adding investment decisions.

New sources of cash flow are increasingly hard to find. In an environment of constrained payment, scarce resources, and increased competition, the cost of making bad capital investment decisions can be severe. Uninformed or poorly analyzed decisions can have financial and market effects that emerge only three, five, or even ten years later. Such decisions reduce the organization's capital capacity, limiting its ability to pursue future initiatives, and in turn, reducing its ability to achieve or maintain competitive market strength.

The safety net provided in the past by Medicare and Medicaid cost reimbursement and generous indemnity insurance structures no longer exists. Credit market requirements have tightened, demand for new business model investments has increased, and healthcare's operating cash flow and access to affordable capital are constantly challenged. To survive and succeed in the current environment, an organization's capital allocation and management process must be based on principles of corporate finance, including the rigorous and consistent application of solid decision-making criteria, proven quantitative techniques, and enhanced transparency.

THE CAPITAL MANAGEMENT CYCLE

The capital allocation and management process is an integral component of the *capital management cycle*—an organic, circular pathway that defines the flow of analysis and decision making related to the management of capital, as shown in exhibit 1.4. A best-practice capital allocation and management process is the linchpin in an organization's ability to capitalize the strategies that it has defined, quantified, and made operational through the capital management cycle. These strategies, which may be both market based and clinically based and both internal and external, include the following:

- Support for the organization's mission- and community-based imperatives
- Strategic investment in existing service line growth or new businesses and ventures
- Ongoing infrastructure investment in the organization's property, plant, and equipment
- Major and long-term investments, such as partnerships and new outpatient, virtual, or other access enhancements
- Maintenance or growth of balance-sheet cash reserves to fund liquidity levels consistent with optimal access to capital

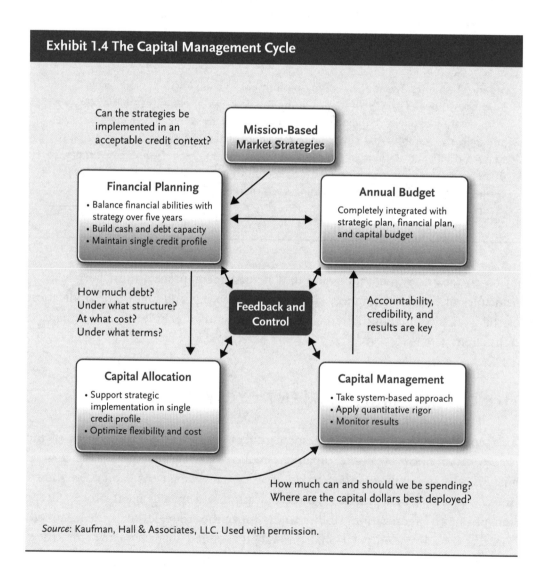

Exhibit 1.4 The Capital Management Cycle

Can the strategies be implemented in an acceptable credit context?

Mission-Based Market Strategies

Financial Planning
- Balance financial abilities with strategy over five years
- Build cash and debt capacity
- Maintain single credit profile

Annual Budget
Completely integrated with strategic plan, financial plan, and capital budget

How much debt? Under what structure? At what cost? Under what terms?

Feedback and Control

Accountability, credibility, and results are key

Capital Allocation
- Support strategic implementation in single credit profile
- Optimize flexibility and cost

Capital Management
- Take system-based approach
- Apply quantitative rigor
- Monitor results

How much can and should we be spending? Where are the capital dollars best deployed?

Source: Kaufman, Hall & Associates, LLC. Used with permission.

Embodying the key concepts of a corporate finance–based management philosophy, the capital management cycle starts with the identification, through the *strategic planning process*, of market- and mission-based strategies that require funding. These strategies define the nature of the organization and the initiatives it wants and needs to pursue in the next five to ten years to achieve its objectives.

In the next cycle stage, the *financial planning process*, the organization quantifies the broad capital requirements and potential effects of the defined strategies. The goal of financial planning is to evaluate whether the identified strategies can be implemented within an acceptable credit context. In conjunction with the financial plan, *capital structure management* focuses on optimizing the use of external sources (e.g., debt and philanthropy, where available) to fund the identified strategies in a manner that ensures maximum flexibility and the lowest possible cost of capital.

The prioritization of specific capital investment opportunities is an iterative step in the capital management cycle that occurs through an organization's *capital allocation process*. Capital allocation balances strategic opportunities with financial capabilities. It ensures that capital is deployed to meet the organization's strategic imperatives while enhancing the organization's financial integrity through its portfolio, as described earlier.

The *annual budgeting process*, which creates a current-year implementation and operating plan, integrates the targets of the strategic and financial plans with the specific investment decisions of the capital allocation process. The annual operating budget should be a strategic document that reflects the operating plan for an organization's base business and implementation of selected strategies. It also provides a means to monitor revenue, expenses, and capital on an ongoing basis.

Capital allocation is thus integrally linked with the organization's strategic, financial, and capital planning processes, as well as its annual budgeting process.

The key principle underlying a successful capital management cycle is as follows:

> Financial performance must be sufficient to meet the cash flow requirements of the strategic plan and, at the same time, maintain or improve the financial integrity of the organization in a carefully evaluated credit and risk context. (Kaufman 2006)

Healthcare executives of not-for-profit organizations vary in their awareness and application of this core principle. Executives who fail to see the interconnectedness of strategy, financial planning, and capital allocation are at significant risk of damaging their organizations' financial performance and continued financial integrity.

TRADITIONAL AND EMERGING, YET PROBLEMATIC, APPROACHES TO ALLOCATING CAPITAL

Approaches to allocating capital vary considerably in contemporary healthcare organizations. A brief look at some common and emerging approaches that are *not* best practice nor recommended can be instructive.

First Come, First Served and Political Approaches

Perhaps the most prevalent approach to allocating capital in healthcare is the *first come, first served approach.* In hospitals and health systems that use this approach, specific projects are evaluated in a serial fashion as they arise throughout the calendar year.

Organizations that employ this approach often go to great lengths to calculate the total amount of cash flow available to be spent on capital, which is clearly a best-practice concept. However, as the fiscal year progresses and projects are approved one by one, capital is apportioned against the calculated limit. Inevitably, at some point during the year, a capital request to fund a project or projects capable of bringing significant growth to the organization works its way forward to be approved. Unfortunately, all of the capital may already have been spent, denying (or at best, deferring) funding for a key strategy. The serial nature of initiative evaluation and approval precludes the ability to construct a portfolio of investments with the best overall strategic and financial return. Exhibit 1.5 illustrates how this occurs.

A purely subjective or *political approach* also is problematic. The department, service, or other unit that demands the most gets the most. The trouble is that squeaky wheels with newly applied capital grease do not always bring the best returns. By essentially ignoring quantitative evaluation, this approach assumes that the core business can generate sufficient cash flow on an ongoing basis to support investment initiatives that may not have acceptable returns. Often, this type of process exists in organizations with highly centralized decision making and a culture that uses allocation of capital to reward past behavior or to appease a powerful political constituency.

History-Based and Balanced Scorecard Approaches

Another approach organizations often use is the *history-based allocation approach*, in which capital is allocated the same way it was allocated in the previous year. If a

Suppose that the leaders of an organization have $10 million to allocate to projects during a one-year period. Project A, costing $4 million, is proposed in February, looks good, and is approved. Project B, costing $3 million, is proposed in March, looks acceptable, and is approved. Then Project C arrives in June. It has the best projected return of all three projects and is associated with a key strategic initiative, but it carries a $5 million price tag.

Having already spent $7 million on Projects A and B, the organization simply does not have the funds for Project C. Management is faced with a devil's alternative. Had all three projects been evaluated simultaneously, the leaders would have decided to pursue Projects A and C and to hold off on B. Now the available options are to either forego a strategic opportunity or use precious cash reserves to over-fund capital during the current fiscal year. This situation occurs simply because the business plan for Project C took 60 days longer to prepare than did the plans for Projects A and B.

Source: Kaufman, Hall & Associates, LLC. Used with permission.

hospital's radiology department or a hospital in a multihospital system received $X million or X percent of the total capital dollars this year, it would expect to receive the same (and maybe even an increased number of dollars or a similar percentage) next year. The problem is that in today's rapidly changing healthcare environment, past performance is not always the best predictor of future results, and the focus of past investment may be inconsistent with the organization's current strategic direction.

Some healthcare organizations use a *balanced scorecard approach*, which may evaluate potential investments based on qualitative market and management issues, such as community needs or physician satisfaction. For example, if a proposed project is designed to meet the qualitative goal of enhancing physician satisfaction, the balanced scorecard approach gives it high marks. Often, no quantification is provided.

Corporate finance–based allocation of capital would force the analysis to go a step further and quantify the potential impact of increased satisfaction. Will greater physician satisfaction lead to more effective use of hospital services? If so, what financial impact can be expected? Will ancillary service utilization change, and if so, by what amount? Clearly, the answers to these questions often will be estimates, but even estimates provide the organization with some measure of the investment's potential impact. Qualitative factors must be properly quantified and evaluated within an overall context of performance.

An additional problem with the balanced scorecard approach is its formulaic use of multiple, weighted criteria that essentially codifies the subjectivity of the group responsible for establishing the weightings. For example, if there are ten criteria, it is possible that only 10 percent of the decision weighting would be assigned to financial return—one of the ten criteria. No organization can survive in the long run if it consistently pursues a series of investment decisions that are strategically driven to the detriment of the organization's financial position. Financial return must be weighted more heavily than other criteria, and the portfolio of investments selected must bring a positive return.

Rolling Capital Approach

Some organizations are considering or are using a *rolling capital approach*. This approach attempts to adopt a method successfully used in operating budget management. It is based on the belief that application of regular updates to the organization's operating forecast (e.g., monthly or quarterly) will enable the organization to more nimbly and effectively adjust its capital spending levels and priorities. In its purest form, the rolling capital approach should result in a capital spending plan that would continuously reflect changes in operating performance, new technologies, short-term market reactions, and management priorities.

While this approach can create significant decision-making flexibility, it is not recommended because of its failure to apply key corporate finance principles that are the foundation of the recommended best-practice process, as described later in this chapter and in chapter 2. These key principles include the following:

- **Standardized decision making.** A key component of the rolling capital approach is the aggregation of different types of capital projects into multiple portfolios. For example, project groups might include those focused on financial margins, organizational mission, maintenance, value, cost reduction, and others. Each of these groups is handled differently based on its unique characteristics. This differential handling undermines the organization's ability to provide the standardized decision-making approach that has been shown to be vital to a successful capital allocation process.
- **Project return.** The rolling capital approach applies different return requirements to different project groups based on their intent (e.g., value creation, cost reduction) rather than a common return requirement that is then adjusted for potential risk (see chapter 6). The lack of a common return requirement creates significant opportunity for the process to be manipulated through definition of project types or intent and alternative return requirements. This undermines the integrity of the decision-making process.

- **Portfolio return.** A continuously changing capital spending plan essentially creates serial capital review and approval, which diminishes the organization's ability to understand the potential return on investment of the capital investment portfolio.
- **Corporate-based financing decisions.** The lack of a firm capital portfolio diminishes the ability of the chief financial officer (CFO) to make valid financing decisions. If the portfolio changes, financing structure and cost of capital are affected. A basic tenet of corporate finance is the separation of project and financing decisions. This concept reflects the need to optimize access to capital by matching the organization's approved capital requirements to potential means of financing (i.e., debt versus equity). Furthermore, in the realm of tax-exempt financing, debt must be associated with specific, appropriate capital initiatives with quantified useful lives. If an initiative is altered to reflect a short-term change in priorities, the tax-exempt status of debt issued for the initiative could be materially affected.

As other approaches to capital allocation and management are developed over time, they also should be evaluated relative to current best practices. It is vital to understand whether proposed new approaches embody the key tenets of corporate finance; reflect the reality of capital acquisition and financing in healthcare; and support consistent, standardized, and metrics-based decision making that creates accountability and transparency.

CHARACTERISTICS OF A BEST-PRACTICE PROCESS

The recommended approach to allocating capital in healthcare organizations should be no different than that used by many *Fortune* 500 corporations. A best-practice approach has the following objectives:

- To support the mission and strategic goals of the organization
- To match capital availability to financial performance
- To protect or create capital capacity
- To provide uniform criteria for project evaluation
- To maximize transparency and, therefore, accountability
- To maintain the highest possible bond rating (i.e., optimal access to capital)
- To ensure consistent investment in the highest-performing assets

Structurally, best-practice capital management is founded on the following key elements:

- A high level of governance, education, and communication
- A coordinated calendar and planning cycle
- Direct links to a sound strategic and financial plan
- Clear definitions of available capital and capital expenditures
- Rigorous, quantified, and consistent business planning for each investment opportunity
- A standardized, one-batch review of potential investments
- Consistent application of quantitative analysis using corporate finance–based techniques
- Data-driven and team-based decision making
- Rigorous postapproval project monitoring and measurement

All of these characteristics, which shape the contents of the rest of this book, are evident in leading US hospitals and health systems. In many other organizations, progress is being made and pieces of this best-practice process are in place, but they are not yet fully integrated with the entire process or with the other components of the capital management cycle. In yet other organizations, the problematic approaches described earlier result in varying degrees of dysfunction in the management of the organization's capital process and the results it generates.

An ongoing survey of capital management approaches employed by health systems of varying sizes and locations indicates that most systems have processes with similar characteristics, though with some variations as a result of organizational and cultural characteristics (Sussman 2016). Rigor, discipline, transparency, and standardization are present in all systems that consider their capital allocation and management process to be successful.

Common Challenges

Three significant challenges prevent comprehensive application of important principles and practices related to capital allocation and management:

1. **Overconfidence.** Some executives may believe that because their organization already employs many best-practice components (e.g., use of standardized analytics by designated capital committees to review proposals for individual capital projects), nothing needs to change. However, a best-practice capital

management process requires comprehensive implementation of *all* the key components. Even if an organization generates superior project-based analytics, the annual review and allocation of capital using a single-batch approach, as discussed in chapter 6, is vital. This approach prevents an organization from mistakenly approving a reasonable but mediocre project in the first quarter of the year, only to find itself without capital resources to invest in a more deserving opportunity in the third quarter. Furthermore, in this type of serial approval scenario, the organization cannot know the true value of the total portfolio of capital decisions made on a fiscal-year basis until well after the fact.

2. **Politics and management style.** The management style of some leaders can prevent the development and use of a best-practice process. Some CEOs and CFOs find it easier to make unilateral capital decisions than to deal with the politics of a process. They may not want to involve certain constituencies who have favorite projects. In excluding these stakeholders, however, the leaders exacerbate organizational politics while defining themselves as the lightning rods for other capital decisions that have bad consequences. They do not realize that physicians, patients, board members, community members, department managers, and payers can be effective advocates, not just obstacles.

3. **Perceived financial strength.** An organization's perceived financial strength is perhaps the most pernicious of the three common challenges, especially during times of business model change. Leaders of organizations that have achieved strong performance under a volume-based system may believe that a "bureaucratic" structure for managing capital spending is not needed as the organization moves to a population health, value-based delivery system. This perception, whether the result of overconfidence or lack of focus, leaves many otherwise high-performing organizations vulnerable both strategically and financially. Over several fiscal years, inconsistent capital decisions that are not integrated with an organization's overall strategy can transform a cash-rich entity with a high credit rating into a cash-poor entity with a lower credit rating. The organization will face significant pressure to rebuild its balance sheet while also trying to find dollars to pursue strategic capital needs.

A best-practice approach to capital allocation and management has a framework with four elements: (1) objectives; (2) principles; (3) process governance; and (4) connected, calendar-driven planning and decision making. These four elements are discussed in chapter 2.

IMPLEMENTATION CONSIDERATIONS

Redesigning the capital allocation and management process is a significant change initiative. To achieve an organization's vision, knowing where the journey begins is just as important as knowing where it is going. To understand the organization's starting point, ask the following questions:

- What investments are receiving capital resources in the organization? Are the initiatives receiving resources consistent with the organization's strategies? How has this evolved from traditional areas of focus?
- Which approaches to decision making regarding capital investments have been employed in the organization?
- What, if any, best-practice characteristics are part of the organization's existing capital allocation and management process?
- What challenges might the organization encounter in reevaluating its process?

REFERENCES

Kaufman, K. 2006. *Best-Practice Financial Management: Six Key Concepts for Healthcare Leaders*, 3rd ed. Chicago: Health Administration Press.

Sussman, J. H. 2016. *Survey of Capital Allocation Approaches in 26 U.S. Health Systems*. Skokie, IL: Kaufman, Hall & Associates, LLC.

CHAPTER 2

Establishing the Framework

THIS CHAPTER PROVIDES guidance on establishing a framework to support a best-practice capital allocation and management process.

Establishing this framework typically does not start from ground zero. For most hospitals and health systems, redesigning the capital allocation and management process involves layering new structures, systems, and tools onto existing processes and culture and enhancing their integration. The goal of redesign is to effectively manage the continuously evolving range of capital decisions required under today's new business model, as well as under models of the future.

To highlight practical applications of such concepts, this chapter includes an example of how Avera Health recently redesigned its capital allocation and management process. Exhibit 2.1 describes Avera Health in brief.

FRAMEWORK BASICS

A best-practice approach to capital allocation and management involves the application of a structured, rigorous, and disciplined business process to ensure that the organization remains focused on its true mission and vision. Through this process, capital decision making becomes an organizational function rather than being vested in only one or a few senior executives. Availability of capital is driven objectively and formulaically, not on the basis of subjective management decisions.

Implementing a comprehensive process often involves substantial organizational change. Accordingly, developing the process requires a strong foundation, which must be established by an organization's board of directors and senior executives. The foundation must be consistent with the organization's basic

Avera Health is a faith-based regional health system based in Sioux Falls, South Dakota. Through six regional centers and more than 16,000 employees, Avera Health serves a population of nearly one million residents in South Dakota and surrounding areas of Minnesota, Iowa, Nebraska, and North Dakota. It has 33 hospitals; more than 200 primary and specialty care clinics; 40 senior living facilities; and home care, hospice, and other facilities distributed over a geographic footprint of 72,000 square miles and 86 counties.

Through services provided by nearly 900 clinicians, Avera had 1.73 million clinic visits and 1.17 million outpatient visits in 2016. Gross patient and resident revenue that year was $3.7 billion, and the net profit margin for investment in future services, technology, and capital projects was approximately $44.8 million. Avera is rated A1 by Moody's Investors Service and AA– by Standard & Poor's.

Source: Avera Health. Used with permission.

---

culture and be supported at the highest levels of the organization for increased discipline and structure.

The successful framework that Avera Health developed and implemented includes four elements: (1) objectives, (2) principles, (3) process governance, and (4) calendar-driven planning and decision making.

A New Allocation Framework for Avera Health

In the early 2010s, Avera Health's leaders sought to establish a uniform capital allocation process and related methodology that would provide a "system view" of capital investment. While each of Avera's six regions individually had solid capital allocation processes, the processes were not consistent. Moreover, an avenue for funding broad, system-based strategic initiatives was not available. Each region essentially managed its own capital resources and needs; spending was not connected to the system's overall requirements for growth and evolution.

The goal of redesigning the process was to develop a structure and discipline that would allow for greater transparency and enable systemwide alignment of capital allocation decisions with Avera's broader strategic goals. This structure would ensure that capital would be invested where the system needed it most.

These factors were increasingly important as Avera looked for growth opportunities, including expanding and acquiring new hospitals. Avera's leaders asked questions such as, What corporate-wide initiatives are required to provide care and receive payment under a population health–focused, value- and risk-based business model? How do we invest in our current regions, in new regions, and in non-acute care? Specifics of the redesign process are described later in this chapter.

OBJECTIVES

The first building block of the capital allocation and management process recommended in this book is leadership's development and implementation of formal, clearly articulated, and broadly communicated process objectives or requirements. The objectives may be part of a larger policy statement or appear as a separate document.

At the highest level, an organization's statement of objectives establishes the need for the process design to achieve the following:

- Consistency
- Standardization
- Reliance on analytics
- Known timing
- Accountability
- Integration with the capital management cycle
- Transparency of governance and decision making

Exhibit 2.2 provides sample objectives from capital management processes that were successfully implemented in hospitals and health systems nationwide. Some of these objectives might seem obvious, but they must be articulated nonetheless.

One of these sample objectives, ensuring "that the portfolio of major investment decisions will add measurable financial and strategic value to the organization," introduces two key best-practice requirements. The first is to create a portfolio of capital decisions, which requires evaluating multiple, competing opportunities all at the same time, not serially over the course of several months. For many organizations, this concept represents a fundamental process change.

The second best-practice requirement is for the organization to connect the strategic evaluation of potential opportunities with their financial evaluation. Organizations cannot make valid decisions in a strategic vacuum based solely on potential financial returns. Conversely, project decision making cannot be based on strategic implications of the selected projects without evaluating their related financial implications.

Exhibit 2.2 Objectives of Best-Practice Capital Management

- Provide rational and consistent guidelines for investment decisions.
- Develop uniform criteria and a formal review process for evaluating all investment decisions.
- Align the long-range strategic, financial, and related operating plans of the organization.
- Ensure that the portfolio of major investment decisions will add measurable financial and strategic value to the organization.
- Integrate the financial requirements of the capital management process and operating impacts of approved capital expenditures with the annual budget and multiyear financial plan.
- Enhance the financial strength and integrity of the organization by increasing its capital capacity and maintaining or improving its credit rating.
- Delineate clear roles, responsibilities, and accountability related to capital management and investment throughout the organization.

Source: Kaufman, Hall & Associates, LLC. Used with permission.

The objective articulated earlier in this section establishes the imperative for integrated strategic and financial planning and analysis, one of the most important attributes of a well-designed capital allocation and management process.

Avera Health's Objectives

In addition to the sample objectives outlined in exhibit 2.2, key objectives outlined by Avera Health's system leaders included establishing a process that was highly integrated with system and regional strategies and operating budgets, increasing the transparency of systemwide decision making, and providing enhanced and meaningful opportunities for decision-making input from all major Avera constituencies (e.g., local boards, physicians, management).

PRINCIPLES

To ensure that the capital allocation and management process reflects the organization's core values, a set of principles should be established that govern the design, implementation, and ongoing operation of the process. The principles indicate how the process will achieve the established objectives. Exceptions to the established principles will result in a slippery slope of decision making that could diminish the organization's financial integrity.

Well-articulated principles answer questions such as, How do executives ensure that the process design appropriately incorporates the portfolio concept? What mechanisms will ensure that individual projects and portfolios of projects benefit from integrated strategic and financial analyses? Such principles must be articulated and agreed upon up front by the governing body.

Exhibit 2.3 provides a selected list of principles that have been developed and used by organizations with some of the most successful capital allocation and management processes in healthcare today, including Avera Health. The following sections describe the categories of principles and the topics covered in those categories.

Equal Access to Dollars

The first principle in this category states that all cash generated in the organization will be consolidated and available to meet all needs in the organization and its component entities.

For multihospital health systems—which, like Avera Health, include hospitals, physicians, and other entities that require differing levels of capital—this is a key, if not the most important, principle. Entities that produce more of the capital may prefer an approach that allocates capital based on each entity's contribution to the total dollars available for spending. However, as this principle indicates, *where* the cash flow is generated should not drive access to capital.

The guiding rationale is as follows: We are a system, and all dollars generated in the system should be managed for the benefit of the entire system.

For community hospitals, this rationale means that all departments, programs, or services in the hospital will have equal access to available dollars. Projects originating in departments that do not typically generate high revenues will have equal access to the total dollars available for spending.

At Avera Health, for example, executives determined that all cash flow generated throughout the system should be owned by the system rather than by individual regions. This approach allows the available cash flow for capital to be shared among all entities to generate maximum strategic and financial benefit for the system as a whole. For example, funds might be transferred for a physician alignment opportunity in a smaller region, even if that region's internally generated capital capacity could not support the total investment.

The second principle in this category states that all projects must be considered candidates for available funds. Even though a facility in a health system or a

Exhibit 2.3 Capital Management Process Principles

Equal Access to Dollars

- Establish centralized ownership of all cash flows generated throughout the organization.
- Mandate that all entities and projects have access to those cash flows.
- Consider all projects equally, regardless of origin in the organization.
- Retain centralized ownership of any unspent proceeds, and reallocate available dollars as a centralized function.

Standardized Analytics, One-Batch Review, and Portfolio Decision Making

- Quantify and articulate the strategic and financial benefits of all capital investments.
- Apply an annual, one-batch evaluation process to support portfolio development.
- Separate project evaluation from anticipated funding or financing source, including philanthropic support.
- Establish the need for the approved project portfolio to have a positive net present value, with individual project flexibility.
- Apply a consistent, formulaic basis for allocating any funds that will be managed on a decentralized basis.

A Governed and Strategic Decision-Making Process

- Establish the direct connection between the quality of the financial planning process and that of the capital allocation and management process.
- Include and integrate major acquisitions in both the capital allocation and management process and the organization's long-range strategic and financial plan.
- Establish a complete business plan–based review of capital requests above a certain dollar threshold.
- Mandate that investment decisions related to high-dollar threshold projects be measured and balanced to ensure the organization's ongoing financial strength.
- Define the process for managing multiyear projects, including multiphase planning, review, and approval.
- Require measurement of actual project results against projections to ensure the integrity of the process and the transfer of knowledge.

Source: Kaufman, Hall & Associates, LLC. Used with permission.

department in a community hospital may be losing money, its proposed projects will be considered. Allocation decisions are based on a potential project's fit with the organization's strategic plan and the project's individual merits, not necessarily on past or present performance of the recommending entity.

Standardized Analytics, One-Batch Review, and Portfolio Decision Making

The principles in this category are based on the understanding that standardized quantification of the potential costs and benefits of investment opportunities, as well as simultaneous review of all projects as a portfolio of opportunities, are critical to high-quality decision making. Informed decisions are data-driven decisions. The capital allocation and management process must assume, as a fundamental premise, that the strategic and financial benefits or burdens of any capital investment can be quantified.

Use of standardized analytics, including templates or uniform formats, ensures true comparability of projects, decision-making transparency, and objectivity of a capital management governance group's decisions. When standardized analytics are used, other managers in the organization will know the strategic and financial impact of selected investments, and they also will understand why those that were not selected required more complete explanation (and scrutiny). The result is an improved allocation decision-making process that more directly supports the organization's strategies.

The significant benefits of one-batch, one-time-per-year allocation of capital include governance of the process, control of total capital dollars spent, and enhanced ability of management to ensure consistency of capital investments with overall strategic direction. When dollars are allocated on an ongoing, serial basis, the approval process is piecemeal, too. The result is often approval of projects that compete strategically or create an unacceptable overall risk profile for the organization. Serial decision making also increases the possibility that the capital allocation and management process is a political one.

One-batch capital allocation and portfolio management may represent a fundamental change in the way many organizations allocate and manage capital. Executives and managers may not be accustomed to presenting all their projects at one point in time each year. Thus, managers at hospitals and health systems commonly object to implementing a best-practice process because it requires them to wait for their projects to be reviewed, perhaps up to a full year.

However, one-batch allocation enables the organization to look at the big picture, on a portfolio basis, thereby expanding the field to include projects for which allocation of dollars might not otherwise be considered. For example, an organization identified and tentatively selected a portfolio of six initiatives expected to generate a solid financial return. The total anticipated return may be strong enough to enable the organization to include in the portfolio a seventh or eighth project that will contribute significantly to meeting community needs even though it will not bring the level of return expected for the other six projects.

The big-picture perspective provided by portfolio decision making also enables organizations to review whether the projects in the portfolio represent the right mix from a strategic or market standpoint. For example, suppose an organization has established a strategic objective to increase consumer access to healthcare by developing outpatient facilities in specific geographic markets. Prior to employing portfolio-based decision making, review of individual projects would have resulted in most, if not all, spending being focused instead on hospital campus needs or initiatives in only one market because of the potential returns of the individual projects.

Thus, the strategy to provide increased ambulatory access becomes disconnected from actual implementation through the capital allocation and management process. In this example, a portfolio of capital initiatives could easily be reconfigured to more consistently address the organization's strategic imperatives. Such is not the case if capital decisions are made serially because the organization will not know the totality of its capital investment until after it is spent.

A Governed and Strategic Decision-Making Process

The principles in this category establish the strategic nature of allocating capital and the integral connection between the strategic and financial planning processes and the capital allocation and management process, as described in chapter 1. Without developing a strategic plan and the related financial plan that quantifies the defined strategies' capital requirements and potential effects, the organization will not be able to determine which capital investment opportunities should be pursued.

Process governance, as described in the next section, ensures that decisions are made in a best-practice manner and that selected initiatives are implemented, monitored, and measured against business plan projections. As described more fully in chapter 8, when the capital required for an approved project is less than that originally anticipated, unspent proceeds are returned to the general pool of funds for reallocation by the governance group.

PROCESS GOVERNANCE

Governance is the linchpin to the ongoing consistency, integrity, and success of a capital allocation and management process. Articulated objectives and principles establish the foundation for a high-quality process; design of the governance structure is among the first implementation decisions related to those objectives and principles. This governance structure must be consistent with the established framework.

Process Redesign

To identify the most appropriate governance structure, organizations typically create a steering committee that includes a broad range of the organization's management constituents and mandate that the committee design or redesign the capital allocation and management process. The committee should be charged with reviewing the existing approach to capital allocation and management; assessing its strengths and weaknesses; and defining a truly objective, structured process with the elements described in this book.

Because allocating capital is a management process, the committee should not include board members. The committee may, in fact, be more productive if its membership is based on organizational knowledge and technical capability. Members should bring to the design effort practical knowledge of existing systems and processes, including financial management, materials management, operations, clinical management, technology management, and strategic decision-making processes and capabilities.

In multihospital systems, the committee should include members with both corporate and operating-entity perspectives. In all organizations, it is important to include a committee member who will encourage focus on the organization's mission, vision, and values. The job of the design committee is formidable, representing major organizational change. Creating the right process governance structure with the right participants is vital.

Governance Structure

For a best-practice process to be implemented successfully, the process's roles, responsibilities, and accountabilities must be clearly defined. Although governance structures will vary from organization to organization, governance must involve high-level corporate and operational management. Managing capital is a management process that involves money; through the distribution of dollars, the process also apportions organizational influence and power.

Exhibit 2.4 outlines the distinct role of the board, which should be to provide appropriate oversight of the process (as it does with other management processes, such as financial planning and operational budgeting) rather than being directly involved.

Whether local or systemwide, boards have fiduciary responsibility to protect and enhance their organization's financial resources. They must provide oversight that ensures these resources are used for legitimate purposes and in legitimate ways. The Governance Institute has identified specific practices that are part of a board's core strategic and financial responsibilities. Practices that affect capital allocation and management include the following:

- Articulating a vision and mission for the organization
- Overseeing organizational strategy and strategic planning, which involves review, approval, and monitoring of progress toward specified goals
- Ensuring alignment and integration of all plans (financial, capital, operational, quality improvement, and more) with the organization's overall strategic plan and direction
- Establishing key financial objectives that relate to goals and mission
- Overseeing the thorough and timely development and implementation of capital and operating budgets so that resources are allocated and managed effectively across competing uses
- Ensuring levels of financial performance that support strategic investment and meet established credit goals
- Approving the organization's capital and financial plans and reviewing information on the organization's performance against those plans
- Ensuring prudent investment of excess funds and access to debt and other capital sources

Source: Adapted from Peisert (2013, 2015). Used with permission.

When establishing the governance structure for the capital allocation and management process, an organization should consider the following questions:

- Should governance be exclusively composed of senior or corporate management?
- What roles should be played by the board and constituencies such as medical staff and operating-entity managers?
- Who will and will not have voting privileges?
- How often should the governance group meet?
- Will middle management and clinicians interact with the governance group? If so, how?
- What process steps and tasks should the governance group delegate, and to whom?

With so much at stake, process governance must be completely supported by the CEO. Even if the CEO decides not to actively participate in the governance structure (hereafter called the *capital management council*, or *council*), it should be clear that the CEO and the chief financial officer (CFO) are working in close partnership to effect this key decision-making process change. The CEO's unconditional support and leadership help ensure a level playing field among senior executives and help avoid process runarounds, which are more likely to occur without such leadership.

The council should be heavily weighted toward corporate (organization-wide) representation. The decisions this group makes will have significant strategic and financial consequences for the entire organization, not just one constituency or entity. Selecting one initiative over another is an explicit statement of the organization's long-term strategic direction. If the group that governs and drives such decisions is fraught with political infighting or favors one constituency over another, it cannot make appropriate, strategic decisions on a consistent basis.

Exhibit 2.5 provides a suggested governance structure. The group should include key members of the C-suite—for example, the CEO, CFO, and chief operating officer (COO). Strong consideration also should be given to the chief information officer (CIO), chief nursing officer (CNO), and chief medical officer (CMO), as

---

Exhibit 2.5 Sample Capital Management Governance Structure

Voting Members	Nonvoting Staff Support
• Chief executive officer • Chief operating officer • Chief financial officer • Chief nursing officer • Chief information officer* • Chief medical officer • Operational representatives (two or three members) • Physician or clinical representatives (two or three members)	• Finance staff • Strategic planning staff • Information systems staff • Physician or other provider network development and management staff • Managed care contracting staff • Business development staff • Quality or patient experience staff

*For some organizations, the CIO and additional clinician representatives may not be appropriate as voting members of the capital management council. However, these disciplines should be available to provide analytical and contextual support to the council when needed.

Source: Kaufman, Hall & Associates, LLC. Used with permission.

---

well as newer roles—such as chief transformation officer, chief experience officer, and chief population health officer—and operational executives. For some organizations, additional physician representation beyond the CMO may be appropriate.

In a multihospital system, operational executives typically include CEOs of subsidiary entities or regional executives. In an academic medical center, to tighten the strategic and financial connection between hospital and university operations, the operational executives may include representatives from the faculty practice plan and the academic departments in the medical school. In a community hospital, vice president–level executives responsible for major operating components, such as network management and quality management, may be included as voting members of the governance group.

Some hospitals and health systems include their CIO or lead information systems executive as a voting member of the council; other organizations ensure integration of the CIO's input into the process but, because of the size and scope of information technology (IT) investments, do not extend voting privileges to CIOs.

At a minimum, council participation by operational executives is vital to a best-practice capital allocation and management process. These management team members are responsible for the successful implementation of initiatives selected through the process. Their inclusion provides them with a broader organizational or system view of capital-related decision making and facilitates the direct transfer of knowledge about strategic issues and the success or failure of selected initiatives.

In addition, operational executives' participation in peer project review increases process transparency. Peers know the questions to ask and will not accept incomplete or unsound responses from colleagues. They can accurately assess the scarcity of resources and make this information available to peers and their departments. Operational executives' participation in postallocation review of approved projects, as described in chapter 8, forces more credible up-front project planning.

However, when participating on the capital management council, operational executives must understand that they are acting as organizational, not constituency, representatives. A well-designed, transparent decision-making process will reinforce this requirement.

Centralized Versus Decentralized Governance

Governance of the capital allocation and management process varies considerably by organization type. Typically, an inverse relationship exists between centralization of capital decision making and the organization's size and breadth. In the largest type of organization—multistate, multimarket systems—decision-making authority is often more decentralized. Regional executives or executives of market-leading organizations in the system assume significant decision-making authority. This authority is a function of organizational culture and the maturity of the capital allocation and management process in these systems.

Large multihospital systems, especially Catholic hospital systems, have been at the forefront of design and implementation of corporate finance–based approaches to managing capital. Capital management issues are likely to be more material in large systems—the dollars are bigger, the types of requests are more varied and numerous, and the ability to control investment of strategic capital is more diffuse. These factors have compelled large multihospital systems to address capital allocation and management in a manner similar to that of a *Fortune* 100 company, such as General Electric. Their capital decision-making processes are highly decentralized, rely heavily on standardized analytic techniques, and involve the rigorous application of consistent decision-making criteria throughout the organization.

In contrast, decision-making authority in stand-alone community hospitals and small health systems operating in a single market tends to be highly centralized in the C-suite. This centralization likely has more to do with the CEO's and senior management's ability (or desire) to be involved in the project development process from A to Z than with their technical capabilities. The effect of their involvement is highly variable. In some instances, senior management makes project decisions following extensive and thoughtful analyses. In other situations, senior management uses political influence to gain approval of capital initiatives that otherwise would not have been pursued. Regardless of the level of centralization of decision making, corporate management representation is one constant in the process governance structure of all types of healthcare organizations.

At Avera Health, the CFO championed development of Avera's systemwide capital allocation and management process with the full and critical support of the CEO. A multidisciplinary workgroup was formed that included Avera's CEO, CFO, and COO, as well as CEOs and CFOs from each region in the system, among other key stakeholders. The workgroup assessed Avera's total available capital and how best to create appropriate centralized and decentralized access to those dollars. The workgroup designed formula-driven mechanisms to allocate dollars to the regions for them to manage on a decentralized basis. (This is the concept of nonthreshold capital, which is described in more detail in chapter 5.) In addition, the workgroup also defined the structure by which decision making would occur for higher-dollar and systemwide initiatives. (This reflects the concept of threshold-level capital, described in chapter 6.)

Sample Governance Structures

Described here are sample governance structures at a community hospital, a two-hospital health system, and a larger health system.

Community hospital. The capital management council of a community hospital has both voting and nonvoting members. Voting members include the CEO, COO, CFO, CMO, and CNO. Nonvoting members include the CIO and staff from finance, business development and strategic planning, human resources, facilities management, and clinical support.

Two-hospital health system. Located in a single market, the system has a multidisciplinary capital management council composed of senior leaders who participate in all aspects of the integrated strategic and financial planning and capital allocation and management processes. The team includes the CEO, COO, CFO, CNO, CIO, medical directors of the hospitals, and the director of ambulatory facilities. In this organization, the CIO coordinates IT-related initiatives, validating their strategic importance and operational appropriateness. Because the CIO does not specifically propose initiatives, the CIO has voting privileges and provides the council with an objective and informed perspective. Given the organization's breadth of activities, support staff to the council is broad and includes the director of facilities management and the vice presidents of operations, strategic planning, and finance.

Multihospital system. The voting members of the multidisciplinary governance group at Avera Health include the CEO, COO, CFO, CMO, and corporate executive vice president for culture; the chief administrative officer of Avera Medical Group; and three regional CEOs and presidents, who serve three-year terms and are selected by the council chair. Nonvoting staff support is provided by the finance and planning staff; the CIO; the corporate senior vice president of supply chain; and functional experts in such areas as facilities, IT, and equipment.

CONNECTED, CALENDAR-DRIVEN PLANNING AND DECISION MAKING

After establishing the structural framework for decision making and governance, organizations must create an environment that fosters comprehensive capital decision making. Effective allocation of capital requires coordination between the organization's strategic, financial, and capital planning processes and its capital allocation and management and budgeting processes. The timing and structure of these processes should reflect their interdependent nature and be rigorously observed.

Integrated and Portfolio-Based Planning

The process of allocating and managing capital is shaped by the organization's culture. An organization with an embedded planning culture uses capital allocation and management as the means to implement strategies and initiatives defined and developed through its annual planning processes.

An integrated planning cycle ensures that *strategic planning* is completed within the context of the organization's financial capabilities and that initiatives are comprehensively analyzed from both strategic and financial contexts. Annual *financial planning* identifies the required levels of financial performance that ensure funding of selected strategies while maintaining or improving the financial position of the organization at a given level of capital access and risk. The results of the *financial plan* then drive the targets for the annual *operating budget* and define the levels of *capital available for allocation* (see exhibit 2.6). This type of planning requires an integrated and disciplined approach to capital allocation and management that relies, ultimately, on a rigorous portfolio approach to decision making.

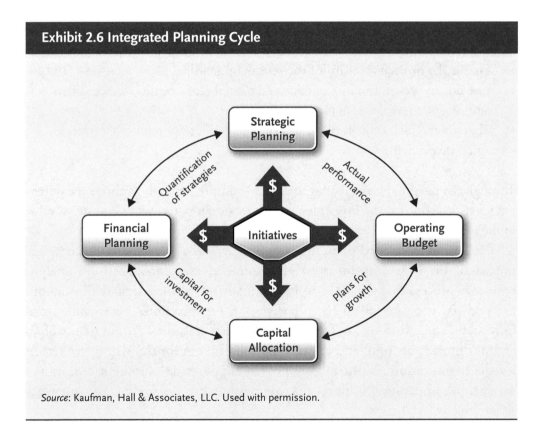

Exhibit 2.6 Integrated Planning Cycle

Source: Kaufman, Hall & Associates, LLC. Used with permission.

Certain portfolio-based questions related to strategic and financial issues should be considered in integrated planning. Strategic questions include the following:

- Should we continue to operate all our current service lines and in all our current markets?
- In which markets or service lines should we invest heavily? In which should we invest at a level solely to maintain services? In which should we reduce investment or divest?
- Are new market or service line investments required to meet our strategic goals for growth?

These questions establish the organization's investment direction, defining the parts of its portfolio (the markets and service lines) targeted for new investment, growth, maintenance, or divestiture.

Financial questions quantify the implications of investment in the strategic portfolio. They include the following:

- What level of overall return is required from our investment in strategic initiatives?
- What is the projected return of the selected portfolio?
- How do changes in the mix of allocated capital (e.g., facility, service line, technology) affect the overall portfolio return?
- What are the cash flow implications of the proposed portfolio of strategic capital investment?

Through the portfolio view, management can comprehensively evaluate the potential for its strategic capital investments to generate short-term and long-term value to the organization.

The goal of integrated planning is to understand and evaluate the complete impact of the organization's strategic capital investments. Portfolio analysis requires a process that allocates capital annually rather than serially throughout the year. By batching all of its initiatives, an organization's management can fully assess the return on investment and annual cash flow requirements of an entire strategic portfolio, and create a portfolio that optimizes risk versus return for the organization. A portfolio approach supports development and implementation of operating budgets that are designed to implement the organization's selected strategies.

The best-practice capital decision-making calendar segregates the fiscal year into two major components of roughly six months each. The first component is the planning component, during which the organization updates and challenges its assessment of its strategic and financial positions. The second component uses the analysis and targets established during the planning component to create annual operating and capital plans focused on implementing the defined strategies.

The Planning Component: From Strategic Planning to Financial Planning

Because of its inherent scarcity, capital must be allocated according to a sound strategic and financial plan, which includes good ideas worthy of investment. If the portfolio of ideas articulated in the plan will not generate the incremental cash flow needed to support the plan's performance requirements, the management team should either go back to the drawing board and identify ideas that will do so or consider alternatives—such as acquisitions, joint ventures, and other types of partnerships—to meet the organization's mission while achieving competitive financial performance.

Effective strategic plans are based on strategic and market realities. Thorough analyses of comprehensive data enable hospitals and health systems to identify financially viable competitive strategies. Numbers in isolation may not tell the story, but the combination of data provides the needed big picture about an organization's performance in its competitive environment. Multiple market and strategic position variables are vital to build the required quantitative fact base. Trends, which show track record and momentum, are important in addition to annual numbers. Key questions that will be answered through ongoing analysis are listed in exhibit 2.7.

Each strategic capital initiative should benefit from the development of a business plan that describes the business or investment concept and its financial effect in significant detail. This plan provides the basic documentation and analysis necessary for a valid capital decision. Exhibit 2.8 outlines the elements vital to business planning, which is described in more detail in chapter 6.

Strategic analysis (including detailed market and competitive assessments) and business planning can and should occur throughout the year, but the strategic and financial plan update must happen at one point in time to initiate the year's planning process. The annual update of the strategic plan provides the starting point for understanding the organization's long-term market objectives and the related strategic capital requirements necessary to reach those objectives.

The financial plan quantifies both how the initiatives identified in the strategic plan update will affect overall volume, revenue, cost, and other financial indicators and what capital will be required to pursue those initiatives (exhibit 2.9). By truly integrating the strategic and financial planning processes, management can establish the short-term and long-term profitability and cash flow targets that will enable the organization to fund its strategy over a specified period.

Exhibit 2.7 Key Questions Asked and Answered During a Strategic Planning Process

- Which areas or regions does the organization currently serve? What is the organization's market share? How has this share changed over time, and how might it change as networks form to manage population health?
- What are the current and projected future characteristics of the population and the local economy?
- What changes are anticipated in the demand for healthcare services in the market? How will changes in the payer and employer environment, demographics, and emerging technologies affect future demand for the inpatient and ambulatory services the hospital provides?
- What is the organization's current service delivery configuration, and what is the condition of its physical assets? How might these change to meet new needs for services in ambulatory and home settings?
- Who are the organization's principal competitors? How are these competitors positioned, and what strategies are they pursuing? How will these strategies affect the organization's position?
- What important trends are occurring in value-based contracting and in inpatient and ambulatory service utilization?
- What is the organization's desired role in population health management? What are its program or service strengths, weaknesses, and development opportunities relative to that desired role?
- What is the structure of the physician market and the organization's physician staff? How might the organization need to develop its physician enterprise for the provision of clinically integrated services in new networks that are forming?

Source: Kaufman, Hall & Associates, LLC. Used with permission.

Exhibit 2.8 Core Elements of Comprehensive Business Planning

- Defining the proposed business or investment and the specific strategic objectives it will address
- Quantifying the capital resources required to initiate, complete, and maintain the proposed investment
- Delineating the potential population to be served and the way that population's health or care needs will be enhanced by the investment
- Projecting the initial and ongoing operating requirements associated with the proposed investment
- Calculating the potential return on investment, including analysis and quantification of key risks associated with the investment
- Identifying potential exit strategies and related performance measures

Source: Kaufman, Hall & Associates, LLC. Used with permission.

Exhibit 2.9 The Planning Component: Key Inputs and Outputs

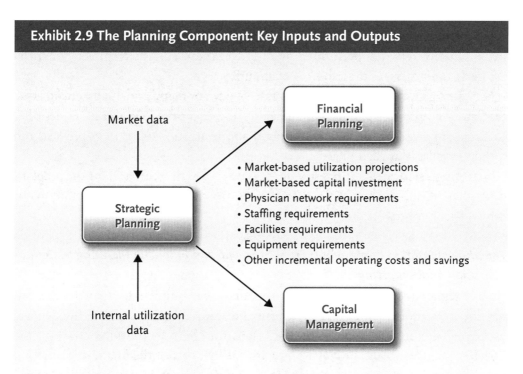

Market data

Financial Planning

Strategic Planning

- Market-based utilization projections
- Market-based capital investment
- Physician network requirements
- Staffing requirements
- Facilities requirements
- Equipment requirements
- Other incremental operating costs and savings

Internal utilization data

Capital Management

Source: Kaufman, Hall & Associates, LLC. Used with permission.

Preplanning for Multiyear, High-Dollar Projects

Because of the high degree of change in healthcare and the need for investment in new capabilities and infrastructure, high-dollar, multiyear projects are increasingly common in hospitals and health systems. The planning phase for these types of projects may extend to several years, so it may be necessary to establish early-stage "waypoints" for allocation decision making. Waypoints include the concept phase and the preplanning phase.

The *concept phase* addresses whether the project makes sense strategically and broadly defines the capital that may be required. It involves activities that are internal to the organization and typically require no material funding.

The *preplanning phase* includes assessing the feasibility of accomplishing the initiative within the defined capital parameters. Specific senior executives (members of a council subcommittee) may authorize activities such as the following:

- Assessing the project's economics at a high level
- Confirming that the project is consistent with the organization's strategic plan
- Confirming that the project is generally safe
- Identifying potential questions regarding the organization's ability to accommodate the project
- Evaluating the likelihood of philanthropic support for the project

This assessment can be funded through a preplanning contingency budget for limited evaluative activities performed by external experts such as architects, financial advisers, and others, as described in chapter 3.

Early-stage evaluation improves strategy development and helps ensure that regulatory needs can be addressed efficiently and effectively. Exhibit 2.10 identifies the scope of activities, resources, required approvals, frequency of approvals, and funding available at each phase.

Creating a separate contingency fund, as described in chapter 3, for the preplanning phase ensures that proposed initiatives are properly evaluated before major capital is committed to them.

The Implementation Component: From Strategic and Financial Planning to Capital Allocation and Budgeting

After integrated strategic and financial planning is completed, organizations can develop and implement annual operating and capital budgets. These budgets are essentially the annual implementation plans for the organization's strategy; the operating budget should be consistent with the first year of the financial plan. That way, all constituencies understand that operating budget constraints are required to ensure the organization's continued ability to access capital to fund its strategies.

Exhibit 2.10 Concept and Preplanning Phases for Multiyear, High-Dollar Projects

	Concept Phase	Preplanning Phase
Scope of activity	Broad definition of costs, strategic fit, and impacts on facility	• Feasibility analysis to detail capital required and impacts on facility • Completed business plan
Resources	Internal resources only	• Outside architects • Organization's finance, planning, and facilities staff
Approval required to enter phase	None	• Capital management council subcommittee
Frequency of approvals	Not applicable	• Continuous on a monthly basis
Funding available	None	• $X per project • $X annually organization-wide

Source: Kaufman, Hall & Associates, LLC. Used with permission.

The operating targets defined in the strategic and financial plan also quantify the amount of cash flow available each year to fund capital. The first-year profitability and cash flow targets or projections from the planning process should be used to calculate the organization's annual capital constraint.

A best-practice capital management process begins by identifying the capital constraint, as described in chapter 3. The *capital constraint* is the maximum amount of cash flow the organization can spend on capital in each year, based on the organization's long-term strategic and financial goals. The capital constraint reflects key management decisions regarding the organization's overall debt structure, the level of required cash reserves, and the profitability required to sustain and enhance the organization's access to capital. Exhibit 2.11 illustrates key implementation inputs and outputs.

Putting It All Together

The beauty of a connected process (exhibit 2.12) is best illustrated when senior executives go to the board for budget approval. Instead of having to field difficult questions regarding levels of profitability, capital, salaries, and other variables, senior executives can present an integrated package. Following is a sample presentation they can make:

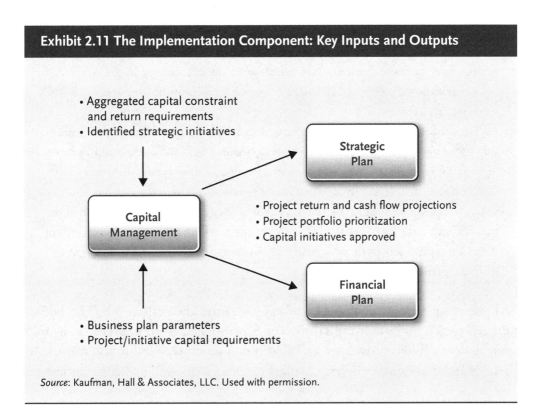

Exhibit 2.11 The Implementation Component: Key Inputs and Outputs

- Aggregated capital constraint and return requirements
- Identified strategic initiatives

Strategic Plan

Capital Management

- Project return and cash flow projections
- Project portfolio prioritization
- Capital initiatives approved

Financial Plan

- Business plan parameters
- Project/initiative capital requirements

Source: Kaufman, Hall & Associates, LLC. Used with permission.

Exhibit 2.12 Disciplined Integration of Organizational Planning

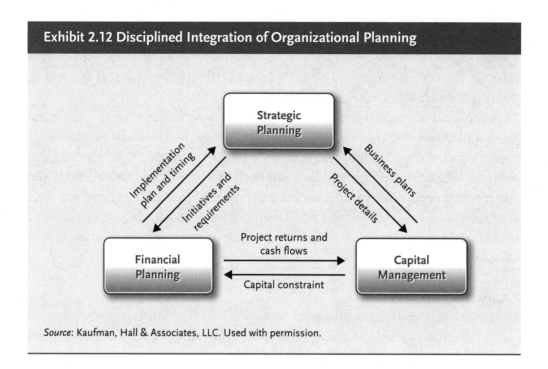

Source: Kaufman, Hall & Associates, LLC. Used with permission.

Here is our overall, *multiyear strategy*, including the specific strategic initiatives anticipated to be implemented in the coming year. Based on this strategy, here is our *strategic and financial plan*, which quantifies the capital and operating requirements of the identified multiyear strategy and associated initiatives; identifies financial performance targets consistent with funding the overall strategy in the context of our organizational credit and risk parameters; and positions us for ongoing, future strategic investment.

Finally, based on those long-term targets and requirements, here are our current-year *operating and capital budgets* that are consistent with the first year of the strategic and financial plan, which is consistent with our strategy, mission, and values. The budgets include our *recommendations for investing capital* to implement the initial initiatives in support of the multiyear strategy. These capital recommendations fit within the budgeted cash flow and minimum cash reserve targets, consistent with our capital constraint as well as our short-term and long-term strategic and financial plan.

Presenting such an integrated package facilitates discussions with the board, rating agencies, and other capital market constituents, as appropriate, at a truly strategic level. It also provides a tool that senior executives and others can use to measure and monitor the success or failure of the strategic and operating initiatives.

Ultimately, the integrated plan offers a finite and quantitative platform from which to launch next year's planning process.

An Integrated Calendar

Organizations with a best-practice, corporate finance–based capital allocation and management process focus significant time and energy on developing and implementing a practical, but highly integrated, planning calendar. Exhibit 2.13 illustrates how the analysis and results of strategic planning, budgeting, capital

Exhibit 2.13 Sequence of Planning and Implementation Activities

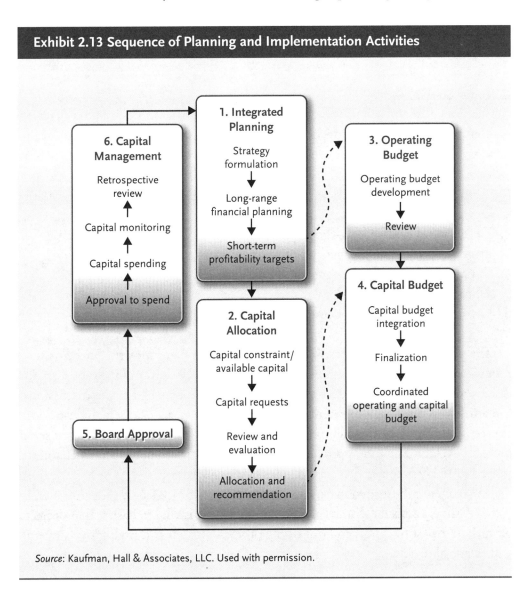

Source: Kaufman, Hall & Associates, LLC. Used with permission.

allocation and management, and approval tie directly to an organization's overall and ongoing decision-making process. The process calendar, as shown in exhibit 2.13, should reflect the integrated flow of the capital management cycle.

From strategic plan development to ultimate capital approval, this decision-making cycle takes a full year to complete. Typically, strategic planning occurs during the first three to five months of the fiscal cycle. Quantification and integration of identified initiatives into the financial planning process occurs during the next two to three months. This leaves four to seven months to complete the annual budgeting and capital allocation and management processes.

Allocation of capital should be scheduled to conclude approximately one month before finalizing the annual operating budget so that management can incorporate the allocated sums and related operating impacts of selected projects into the appropriate departmental operating budget for implementation.

Calendar Components

An integrated calendar helps to ensure efficient, effective, and consistent decision making. Complete integration of planning processes supports seamless decision making. The typical order of events in an annual decision-making calendar is as follows:

1. Develop and update strategic plan
2. Develop and update long-range financial plan
3. Establish profitability targets and the capital constraint
4. Initiate development of operating budget
5. Allocate capital
6. Finalize current-year operating and capital budgets

The process of allocating capital must be an integral component of the organization's overall strategic and financial planning calendar. It should not be a stand-alone process or simply added on to the tail end of operating budget discussions. Organizations often try a different order of process steps, for example, by providing revised strategic plans throughout the calendar year. However, this leads to serial project development and approval problems, such as those described in chapter 1 related to the first come, first served approach to allocation.

The sequence illustrated in exhibit 2.13 is the only process flow that consistently provides superior results. Strict calendar management is vital to ensure that projects or initiatives do not slip in and out of the process without comprehensive strategic and financial review.

Exhibit 2.14 describes the status of the calendar approach at several surveyed health systems at the time of this writing. Suffice it to say that there is significant room for improvement.

Communicating and Maintaining the Calendar

To be truly effective, the calendar of decision-making events must be clearly defined, documented, and communicated throughout the organization. Communication should be ongoing, and all staff should be aware of the date when capital requests and related analyses are due and the date when projects are evaluated.

Due dates for the submission of capital requests and analyses for projects that exceed a dollar threshold defined by the organization—threshold capital projects, as described in chapter 4—must be established well in advance, with little to no tolerance for late submissions. Executives and the capital management council should refuse to consider until the following year any threshold capital projects that are submitted late. It generally takes only one or two such refusals for staff to understand that the dates are hard and nonnegotiable. When the council sticks to its guns, everyone enjoys definite and distinct benefits.

Exhibit 2.14 Status of Calendar Management at Health Systems

A survey of capital management processes in healthcare systems indicates that each system maintains a process calendar that it believes is specific and communicated. Although the systems typically delineate all key process steps, the calendar is often limited to the annual budgeting process component of capital allocation and management. Project allocation and approval occur year-round; only decisions related to departmental capital and capital used to replace existing equipment are governed by the calendar. The calendar also is typically designed as a compliance tool instead of a means for integrating strategic and financial planning, especially in multimarket systems.

The systems adhere to established deadlines to various degrees, depending on their corporate culture, discipline, degree of centralization, and process evolution. For some, the calendar is a significant management tool. For others, the calendar is more theoretical than practical and is essentially unknown outside the CFO's office. The most commonly raised issue is how to fit the process of allocating capital into the annual budgeting process.

Organizations that have stopped reviewing projects serially and now use one-time batch review can readily integrate the capital management process with other processes governed by the calendar.

Source: Sussman (2016).

The appendix table at the end of the chapter shows Avera Health's detailed schedule of activities and responsibilities, which clearly communicates expectations. Developed and maintained by Avera's director of finance, this document integrates long-range financial planning, the operating budget, and the capital budget.

Capital Management Council Schedule

The capital management council should meet one time each year to evaluate capital investment opportunities and make capital allocation decisions for the subsequent year. In addition, the council should meet quarterly to revalidate projects for funding approval, to monitor the progress of funded initiatives, and to evaluate whether contingency funds should be released for emergency or out-of-cycle needs. The timing of the review and approval of threshold capital requests must be early enough in the process calendar to allow sufficient time for annual budget submissions to reflect departmental operating impacts of approved projects. These topics will be addressed more fully in chapters 5 through 8.

Monthly council meetings are unnecessary and unproductive, and they imply that allocation decisions can be made every month, which should not be the case. Conversely, monitoring of capital spending against approved and funded projects should be part of the monthly budget review process and should require variance explanations similar to those provided for the operating budget. At its quarterly meetings, the council can review the status of capital projects with variance issues.

As discussed in chapter 9, hospitals and health systems may wish to consider making the transition to a calendar system over a multiyear period, because the scope of changes that are required is typically extensive. Exhibit 2.15 provides a sample integrated planning schedule that incorporates key capital management activities.

Exhibit 2.16 shows the integrated planning and allocation tasks and time frames Avera Health designed for its capital allocation and management process. In transitioning to this schedule, Avera had three objectives for the capital process:

1. Full integration into Avera Health's overall decision-making processes
2. Timing that would account for the organization's continuous decision-making requirements
3. Support for creation of a "seamless" decision-making process

Avera's council meets quarterly, with a specific agenda for each meeting. The council reviews all threshold capital projects (i.e., high-dollar projects, as described in chapter 4) annually in a single-batch process at the end of its second quarterly meeting.

Exhibit 2.15 Organizing for Calendar Management: Sample (January-to-December Cycle)

To make the transition to an integrated calendar-management system, a two-hospital health system divided its fiscal year (a calendar year) into major management functional periods and assigned each calendar component to a specific council with corporate oversight as follows:

- *Market assessment*, which occurs in November and December—13 and 14 months ahead of the budget year—has oversight from a decision support council composed of key leaders in the market and decision support areas of each hospital.
- *Strategic planning*, which occurs from January through April, has oversight from a strategic planning council.
- *Financial planning*, which occurs from April through September, includes two stages: long-range financial planning, which involves a high-level assessment of the viability of the strategic plan, and identification of the profitability targets and the capital constraint (by June 15), followed by a detailed project-by-project analysis of plan elements and an overall portfolio analysis. Oversight is provided by the decision support council.
- *Capital allocation* culminates with allocation recommendations made to a capital management council on October 1, following the development and analysis of capital requests during the second and third quarters.
- *Operations and capital funding* commences with operating budget development during the third quarter, based on the short-term profitability targets identified during the financial planning process. The capital allocations approved on October 1 are integrated into the operating and capital budgets, finalized, and reviewed/approved by the board on November 15. Hospital/system management oversees this process.

Source: Kaufman, Hall & Associates, LLC. Used with permission.

Strong support from senior administration and broad representation on the workgroup both were critical to the success of Avera's redesign initiative. Having stakeholders intimately involved in developing the process structure increased buy-in to the ultimate look and feel of the process design.

IMPLEMENTATION CONSIDERATIONS

Almost every organization has a concise policy document related to capital decision making. Unfortunately, an organization's formal process often does not fully follow

Exhibit 2.16 Sample Integrated Planning Calendar (July-to-June Cycle)

Task	Timing
Strategic plan development and approval	July to October
Distribution of capital project approval forms	October 1
Development of entity/system financial plan	November to December
Consolidated financial plan complete/five-year targets established	December 31
Submission of nonthreshold capital requests	December 31
Determination of system capital constraint	January 31
Allocation of funds to threshold and nonthreshold capital pools	January 31
Deadline for submission of threshold capital approval forms*	January 31
System capital approval review (including discussions)	February
Complete threshold capital review packages to capital management council	March 15
Capital management council meeting	March 31
Allocation of threshold capital	March 31
Allocated capital incorporated into facility annual budgets and financial plans	April
Corporate review of submitted budgets issue resolution	early May
Corporate review and sign-off	end of May
Board approval of operating and capital budgets	June

*Includes noncapitalized investment decisions (e.g., physician recruitment and program start-up).

Source: Avera Health. Used with permission.

the policy. Of greater concern is the fact that the informal process typically runs counter to the letter and spirit of the formal, expected process.

An organization should consider how its formal and informal processes align with its current policy and its vision for a redesigned process. *Do* and *do not* considerations for effective redesign include the following:

- *Do* assemble a multidisciplinary team of administrators, users, analytic resources, and decision makers to redesign the process.
- *Do* fully evaluate and document the current processes.

- *Do not* be afraid of contrary perspectives on the redesign team. It is better to address differences today than to try to break down barriers after process implementation.
- *Do not* allow redesign to take on a life of its own. A typical redesign can be achieved during four or five sessions of three or four hours each, within a 90-day horizon.

REFERENCES

Peisert, K. C. 2015. *Governing in the New Healthcare Industry: 2015 Biennial Survey of Hospitals and Healthcare Systems.* San Diego, CA: The Governance Institute.

————. 2013. *Governing the Value Journey: A Profile of Structure, Culture, and Practices of Boards in Transition. 2013 Biennial Survey of Hospitals and Healthcare Systems.* San Diego, CA: The Governance Institute.

Sussman, J. H. 2016. *Survey of Capital Allocation Approaches in 26 U.S. Health Systems.* Skokie, IL: Kaufman, Hall & Associates, LLC.

Appendix: Sample Detailed Annual Integrated Planning and Budgeting Schedule

Due Date	Long-Range Financial Plan Discussion Item	Operating Budget Discussion Item	Capital Budget Discussion Item	Responsibility
9/1/15			Avera Regional Presidents and Regional CFOs review potential/preliminary capital projects in excess of $500K over the next 5 years.	Avera COO, Avera Operations Council, and CFOs
10/7/15	Preliminary discussion of revenue assumptions for long-range plan (LRP) for volume and payer categories			Avera CFO, Avera COO, Avera Medical Group Chief Administrative Officer, Avera SVP of Managed Care, and Regional CFOs
10/15/15	Preliminary assumption development for LRP for expense categories			Avera CFO, Avera COO, Avera SVP of Human Resources, Avera VP of Supply Chain, and Regional CFOs
10/28/15	Final assumption development for LRP for volume and expense categories			Avera CFO, Avera COO, Regional CFOs
11/1/15 – 11/26/15		Departmental budgeting software refresher training available		Avera Administrative Council/Avera Finance staff

11/24/15	Review of LRP assumptions; expectation of Avera Central Services (ACS) expense increase	Review of major operating budget system initiatives	Avera CEO, Avera COO, Avera CFO, and Finance staff
12/2/15	Operations Council LRP overall assumption review; CFOs invited to participate	Review of major operating budget system initiatives	Avera Operations Council and Regional CFOs
12/18/15		Budget packets distributed electronically to Avera Administrative Council	Avera Finance staff
1/22/16		Deadline for threshold projects due to Avera within capital management software	Avera Finance staff and Regional CFOs
1/25/16	Final LRPs and capital initiatives list due to Avera from the regions		Avera CFO and Regional CFOs
1/25/16	Consolidation of LRP		Avera VP of Financial Planning
1/25/16	Distribution of materials to Functional Review Teams and Service Lines		Avera VP of Financial Planning
1/25/16–1/31/16		Determination of capital constraint and dollars available of FY 2016 capital	Avera CFO and VP of Financial Planning

(continued)

(continued from previous page)

Due Date	Long-Range Financial Plan Discussion Item	Operating Budget Discussion Item	Capital Budget Discussion Item	Responsibility
1/29/16		Avera departmental budgets due to Finance department		Avera Administrative Council
2/1/16–2/15/16			Functional review meetings for IT, program, facility, and equipment	Functional Review Chairs and team members, Avera CFO, VP of Financial Planning
2/15/16			Allocation of funds to threshold and non-threshold capital pools	Avera CEO, COO, CFO, and VP of Financial Planning
2/8/16–2/26/16		Avera budget meetings with members of Avera Administrative Council		Avera Finance staff
2/16/16			Assembly of threshold projects for Capital Management Council and distribution of capital packets to council members	Avera VP of Financial Planning
3/7/16			Completed review of all threshold capital projects due back to Avera Finance department	Capital Management Council

Date			
3/10/16	LRP review with CEO and COO	Draft Avera departmental budget; review with CEO and COO	Avera CEO, COO, Finance staff
3/17/16		Capital Management Council meeting and allocation of threshold capital	Capital Management Council
3/18/16	Reconcile ACS fees with ACS node for 2016 LRP		Avera VP of Financial Planning
3/18/16		Corporate provides regions with final ACS fees, IT cost allocation, Centralized Business Office, marketing, insurance, and any other significant costs	Avera Finance staff and Regional CFOs
3/25/16	Allocated capital incorporated into facility's LRP	Allocated capital incorporated into facility's operating budget	Regional CFOs
3/28/16 – 4/12/16	Files to consultant		Avera VP of Financial Planning
4/12/16		System Members Compensation Committee meeting	System Members

(continued)

(continued from previous page)

Due Date	Long-Range Financial Plan Discussion Item	Operating Budget Discussion Item	Capital Budget Discussion Item	Responsibility
5/14/16		Final proposed hospital operating budgets received at Avera	Final proposed non-threshold capital budgets received at Avera	Hospitals
5/14/16		Analysis of budgets, benchmarks, debt service requirements, and bond indenture compliance to Avera Financial Performance Committee; final proposed capital budgets received at Avera		Avera Finance staff
6/02/16	Review of final strategic plan at Avera Financial Performance Committee meeting	Review of final operating budgets at Avera Financial Performance Committee meeting	Review of final capital at Avera Financial Performance Committee meeting	Avera Financial Performance Committee
6/15/16	Final review and approval of 2016 final strategic financial plan	Final review and approval of fiscal year 2016/2017 operating budgets	Final review and approval of fiscal year 2016/2017 capital budgets	Avera Board of Directors

Source: Avera Health. Used with permission.

CHAPTER 3

Determining the Capital Constraint

A BEST-PRACTICE APPROACH to capital allocation and management is framed by a clear definition of the *capital constraint*, or the net cash flow available for capital spending during a designated period.

This chapter addresses how healthcare organizations should answer questions such as, How much can we afford to spend on capital next year? How much can we afford for the next three to five years? Ultimately, the answers must be driven by the organization's long-range strategic and financial plan. The plan should include operating, financial, and capital projections based on the organization's defined strategies. It should also reflect management decisions regarding the organization's targeted long-term financial structure and optimal access to capital, given a specified level of risk tolerance.

Every organization faces a limitation on available capital resources that is determined by the organization's current level of operations, debt structure, and cash position. To make informed and timely capital allocation decisions, organizations must fully understand the capital constraint. Some organizations start the decision-making process by simply reviewing the previous year's spending levels or income statement—for example, net income plus depreciation or a percentage of total operating revenue. However, because such approaches do not account for changes in the organization's balance sheet that affect cash flow, they provide an incomplete view of capital availability, which can lead to financially detrimental levels of capital spending.

To accurately assess its capital constraint, an organization must consider all sources and uses of funds, including principal payments, working capital changes, and additions to balance-sheet cash reserves.

Each organization is unique and has different sources and uses of capital. Fortunately, the capital constraint calculation can account for all such variations. This chapter includes the following two examples that illustrate this point:

- A four-hospital western health system (WHS) with more than 65 healthcare centers and labs uses its unique endowment as a source of cash flow to support its capital capacity.
- Emory Healthcare, a six-hospital integrated academic healthcare system in Georgia, is the clinical enterprise of the Robert W. Woodruff Health Sciences Center of Emory University. Like many academic healthcare systems, Emory Healthcare transfers funds from its clinical enterprise (capital uses) to support the university's medical school.

CALCULATION COMPONENTS

Financial leaders can begin to determine their organization's capital constraint by asking the following question: What amount of cash flow, from both internal operations and external sources, are we reasonably sure can be generated to support the organization's strategic capital needs over a defined period? The answer should include (1) how much the organization can and should borrow and (2) the level of cash flow it can generate and retain from operations in demanding times.

Leaders at Emory Healthcare, for example, calculate the organization's capital constraint annually. Their calculation incorporates the long-term strategic and financial direction of Emory Healthcare and the university's medical school in the multiyear financial planning process and related development of financial projections. For the consolidated system, the total cash flow available for capital spending is a function of the following:

- Existing cash on hand versus targeted levels
- Projected operating results
- Planned use of external debt, as determined in conjunction with Emory University
- Projected levels of philanthropy not accounted for on the income statement (e.g., capital campaign contributions)

Against the projected cash availability, Emory's strategic and financial plan also defines noncapital uses of cash that apply to the consolidated Emory system, including the following:

- Targeted levels of strategic cash reserves for Emory Healthcare
- Carryforward spending for previously approved projects
- Principal payments required on debt
- Working capital needs
- Transfers to the university and medical school
- Other contingencies

Exhibit 3.1 outlines the basic components of the capital constraint for most organizations. A more detailed look at each component follows.

Cash Flow

Cash flow, the starting point in the calculation of capital availability, is typically determined by adding income and depreciation. However, the definition of *income* can vary from organization to organization. Some financial leaders believe that income should be limited to income from operations; other leaders include all nonoperating sources, such as investment income, contributions, and gains on sale of assets. Therefore, defining income is a significant, initial strategic step in an organization's capital allocation and management process.

Exhibit 3.1 Components of the Capital-Constraint Calculation

Cash flow

Plus total sources of cash	**Less total uses of cash**
Debt proceeds	Working capital
Philanthropy	Principal payments
Other sources of cash	Carryforward capital
Cash reserve requirements	Other uses of cash
	Transfers to outside organizations

= Total cash available for capital

Less contingency

= Net cash flow available for capital allocation—the capital constraint

Source: Kaufman, Hall & Associates, LLC. Used with permission.

By including only operating income in determining its cash flow, an organization creates an automatic reserve to increase balance sheet liquidity at the expense of current-year capital spending. Organizations that adopt this approach typically have a weak balance sheet or a history of spending too much capital. Organizations that include income from all sources in their cash flow calculation maximize their current-year capital availability, but they must establish and meet the rigorous balance sheet cash reserve targets in their strategic and financial plan. While both Emory Healthcare and WHS include operating and nonoperating income in their beginning cash flow determination, many other successful organizations exclude nonoperating income as an additional contingency factor.

Debt Proceeds

This capital constraint component includes proceeds from external debt that are anticipated to be issued in the upcoming years as well as the unspent, but still available, proceeds of debt issued in prior years. An organization should incur no more debt than allowed to maintain a credit rating that enables it to compete in the marketplace and maintain optimal access to capital. The amount of debt the organization can support within a desired credit-rating profile is its *debt capacity*. Access to debt capacity in the form of incremental, new debt is a function of

- creditworthiness, which is a factual analysis performed by agencies that rate healthcare debt; and
- willingness of the capital markets to support an organization's perceived strategy, which is an evaluative process undertaken by institutional and other investors.

Healthcare executives must conduct a rigorous debt capacity analysis before starting their annual capital allocation and management process. Typically, this analysis is part of the organization's strategic and financial planning process. Healthcare executives and trustees should view debt capacity analysis as critical, given the importance of external sources of cash and cash flow to an organization's overall capitalization.

Philanthropy

Many not-for-profit healthcare organizations benefit from ongoing donations generated as a result of their community, academic, or faith-based affiliations. Such donations are categorized as nonoperating revenue on these organizations' income statements. Depending on an organization's definition of cash flow (see the Cash Flow section earlier in this chapter), this revenue source may already be part of the capital constraint calculation.

Extraordinary philanthropy is usually associated with a capital initiative or a capital campaign. This source of cash flow often is not recorded as an income item but flows directly to the balance sheet. Thus, explicitly including such philanthropic funds in the calculation of the capital constraint is critical.

The availability of philanthropic dollars raises many questions. For example, should earmarked, donated funds be considered a capital source or be applied to reduce the cost of the project that attracted the funds? How should an organization handle specific-purpose contributions to an entity or program in its capital allocation and management process?

No matter how executives choose to answer these questions, they must be transparent in reporting the flow of philanthropic dollars. These funds should be identified as a source of cash but designated as available only if the identified project is approved. Executives must fully disclose the total capital risk associated with a potential investment before approval and during the project monitoring stage. Maintaining the integrity of the gift and ensuring that a high-quality investment decision is made are essential.

A major teaching hospital, for example, received a donation for the development of an ambulatory center. The gift was large enough to cover the capital costs of the project, making the project essentially free from a net capital perspective. In some organizations, the capital committee does not have to review a project that does not involve a net capital allocation, so the project simply moves forward. The aforementioned teaching hospital, however, required project review. The capital committee's review revealed that although the generous contribution covered capital costs, the ambulatory center would operate at significant, ongoing annual loss. Therefore, moving ahead with the project could place the hospital at significant financial risk.

Working Capital

An organization that is growing, or whose net current assets are growing, will have material year-to-year needs to fund working capital. These working capital requirements flow through the organization's balance sheet and cash flow statement, but not through the income statement. This means that an organization that determines capital spending by using a percentage of operating income will overlook working capital requirements as a potentially significant use or source of cash.

Principal Payments

Payments of principal on existing and anticipated new debt constitute direct uses of cash that are not accounted for on an organization's income statement. Depending on the amortization structure of an organization's outstanding debt, principal payments could materially affect cash flow available for capital.

As an example, consider a small hospital that, because of limited access to the broader capital markets, has financed its major capital needs through capital leases or state-managed equipment-pool loans. These debt structures often have short amortization periods, meaning the organization might repay 15 percent to 20 percent of the asset value each year. Such substantial payments effectively reduce the organization's net cash flow available for capital. If these payments are not included in its capital constraint calculation, the organization might spend more than it should and undermine its balance sheet integrity.

Carryforward Capital

Carryforward capital is defined as approved capital expenditures that have or will have a multiyear cash flow impact as direct deductions from available cash flow.

Carryforward capital comes from different sources and in different forms. Organizations must quantify the specific types, as described below, and amounts to accurately determine their impact on future cash flow available for capital. Regardless of type, cash outflows related to carryforward capital have been approved and are in process. Therefore, the carryforward capital should be one of the direct deductions from available cash flow.

The three basic types of carryforward capital are as follows:

- **Type 1:** Capital dollars originally committed for approved capital projects with a planned, multiyear implementation schedule
- **Type 2:** Capital dollars required to complete an approved project that has been initiated but whose completion will not occur in the current fiscal year, as originally planned, but in the subsequent fiscal year
- **Type 3:** Capital dollars allocated in the current year to projects or other types of capital requests that have not been initiated at the end of the current fiscal year

Organizations should establish specific policies for funding each type of carryforward capital. Such policies are needed to calculate and manage the current-year capital constraint and to ensure deployment of capital dollars according to the organization's strategic and financial plan.

Type 3 carryforward capital typically generates the most complex technical issues. Such issues include the ability to quantify approved spending that has not yet occurred and the impact of large carryforward amounts on the organization's ability to support future capital initiatives. Type 3 carryforward capital also generates complex cultural issues, including a use-it-or-lose-it approach and concern about the rigor of the organization's project management process. Each organization should evaluate these issues to develop policies that are consistent with its culture and structure.

For example, a hospital might determine its net cash flow available for capital spending based on its long-range strategic and financial plan, applying the following parameters for carryforward capital:

- **Type 1:** The impact of Type 1 carryforward capital will be a direct reduction of the capital management council's calculation of net cash flow available for capital. The specific impact will be based on project updates received at the beginning of the subsequent year's capital allocation and management process. Updates will include information on the remaining capital to be spent on approved projects. Even though projects have been approved and initiated, the council may place them on hold or even terminate them, but only in extreme circumstances (e.g., financial deterioration or change of strategic direction).
- **Type 2:** Similar to Type 1, funding of Type 2 carryforward capital will be managed by the capital management council based on project updates received at the beginning of the subsequent year's capital allocation and management process. Based on the schedule, the council will reaffirm the expected completion dates of projects that have been initiated. Unspent capital from the current year will be carried forward to fund completion of the project unless the project is over budget. If the overrun exceeds a predefined budget variance limit, the council will determine both if the project should continue and the source of the funding required for completion. If the project is affirmed and no capital (approved or contingency) remains, the council may fund the project as carryforward capital in the subsequent year's calculation of net cash available or may require the project to be resubmitted for funding from the subsequent year's capital review process.
- **Type 3:** Approved capital projects that have not been committed via purchase order or other written commitment in the year of approval will not be considered carryforward capital. These projects must be resubmitted to the capital management council for review in the subsequent allocation

year. In some instances, an organization may decide that strategically vital investments, the timing of which can be extremely variable (e.g., physician practice purchases or recruitment), should be specifically excluded from Type 3 carryforward capital and instead be handled as Type 1 carryforward capital.

Exhibit 3.2 summarizes recommended parameters for carryforward capital management and provides different approaches to threshold capital and nonthreshold capital (discussed in more detail in chapter 4).

Cash Reserve Requirements

Through the financial planning process, an organization can identify operating performance and balance sheet targets associated with meeting its capitalization needs while maintaining access to capital within defined credit and risk contexts.

Liquidity—the minimum level of required cash reserves—is a critical balance sheet target. Because of uncertainties associated with healthcare's new business model, as in all times of volatility and higher risk, organizations have increased the amount of cash they retain as reserves. The median level of days cash on hand rose from approximately 149 days in 2004 to 219 days in 2015, according to data published by Moody's Investors Service (2016), one of the three agencies that rate healthcare debt. The rating agencies hold that organizations seeking to maintain the strength of their credit ratings must maintain liquid cash reserves (and communicating to the agencies the intent to do so is recommended). Further, because healthcare organizations need to make investments in the transition to value-based care, particularly investments in risk-bearing insurance products or plans, cash reserves provide an increasingly important cushion against the impacts of such strategies (Wareham 2015).

Similarly, the executive team must define the increase in cash reserves as a priority call on the organization's cash flow. Because operating performance is projected through the financial planning process, executives also should define the targeted amount of generated cash flow to be held as balance sheet reserves and include an increase or decrease in those reserves in their capital constraint calculation. In this way, executives can ensure that the amount of capital to be spent will not jeopardize the organization's ability to maintain balance sheet liquidity appropriate to the level of risk inherent in its strategic direction and initiatives.

When an organization calculates capital availability as a percentage of depreciation or income, it cannot directly account for strategic increases in cash reserves. Consequently, the organization's capital budget is disconnected from its balance

Exhibit 3.2 Carryforward Capital Parameters

	Carryforward Type	Carryforward Allowed?	Parameters
Threshold Capital	Type 1 (Planned multi-year expenditure)	Yes	• Periodic monitoring by capital management council • Ongoing revalidation of allocation as long as total project dollars remain at or below original project estimate • Revalidation of allocation and determination of incremental funding if project cost increase is within established variance parameters • Reassessment of project economics and validation of allocation decision if project cost increase is greater than established variance parameters
	Type 2 (Encumbered, but delayed, single-year expenditure)	Yes	• Revalidation of allocation as long as total project dollars remain at or below original project estimate • Reassessment of project economics and validation of allocation decision if project cost increase is greater than established variance parameters
	Type 3 (Unencumbered and delayed single-year expenditure)	No	• Resubmission to the capital management council as a new request
Nonthreshold Capital	Type 1 (Planned multiyear expenditure)	N/A	
	Type 2 (Encumbered, but delayed, single-year expenditure)	Yes	• Verification from operating-entity management that expenditure level remains at or below budget • Limited carryforward timing (e.g., 3 months)
	Type 3 (Unencumbered and delayed single-year expenditure)	No	

Source: Kaufman, Hall & Associates, LLC. Used with permission.

sheet, and the organization cannot accurately understand the effect of a spending level on its access to capital.

Other Sources and Uses of Cash

This catchall category includes the many other calls on, or contributions to, organizational cash not reflected on the organization's income statement that affect liquidity and cash flow available for capital spending. Typical items may include

- funding of pension- or benefits-related shortfalls;
- transfers to universities or medical schools;
- payouts to unaffiliated organizations, such as joint-venture partners or corporate members; and
- payments received from unaffiliated organizations.

For academic medical centers, capital transfers to the university and medical school are typical uses of cash. Including and properly accounting for the impact of these items in the capital constraint ensures that the ultimate calculation reflects true levels of cash flow available for capital spending.

Contingencies

All healthcare organizations should consider unanticipated capital spending in their capital constraint calculation. Described in more detail in chapter 4, contingency capital—considered "safety valve" capital—is a deduction from the *total* cash flow available for capital spending. The result is the *net* cash flow available for capital spending—the capital constraint.

Two types of contingency funds should be considered: system capital contingency and large-project planning contingency. These types of contingencies are described in the following sections.

System Capital Contingency
The system capital contingency is managed by the capital management council and gives the council flexibility to meet unanticipated needs. System capital contingency dollars are available to meet emergency and out-of-cycle needs or to fund project cost overruns at the council's discretion. In addition, system capital

contingency gives the council a cushion if operating results vary significantly and negatively from the financial plan targets. Thus, if actual operating cash flow is under budget, the council can use the system capital contingency to continue to fund needed capital without negative implications for the organization's financial position. This contingency is typically funded at 10 percent of the total cash flow available for capital spending.

Large-Project Planning Contingency

Large projects may require multiphase planning, and organizations should consider the associated costs in the capital constraint calculation. A planning contingency funds the costs that an organization will incur to develop the initial cost estimates and scope for large, multiyear projects. These projects are threshold capital projects, as described in chapter 4.

This contingency increases a new project's visibility and transparency early in the project's life. As a result, the capital management council can direct resources from initiatives that are low priorities or inconsistent with the organization's strategic direction before significant investment (financial and emotional) is incurred.

For example, WHS set the total amount of contingency dollars available to support its preplanning activities at $500,000, with the amount subject to annual review by the capital management council. A council subcommittee governed the contingency by designating proposed threshold project concepts for which preplanning should be pursued and establishing priorities for funding among the designated project concepts. Only projects approved by the subcommittee were authorized to move from the concept to the preplanning phase, an approach described in chapter 2. The activities that would be funded for use of outside resources included

- quantification of potential volume implications associated with the project investment,
- space and building requirements (e.g., an architectural feasibility analysis), and
- projected capital costs.

The hospital system limited budget support for preplanning activities (funded from the total preplanning contingency of $500,000) to $35,000 per project. All preplanning funds originated from the preplanning contingency pool, regardless of the accounting treatment of the expenditures or the eventual outcome of the project.

Putting It All Together

Exhibit 3.3 illustrates a five-year capital constraint calculation used by a multi-hospital system in line with its strategic and financial plan. The capital numbers reflect the system's financial plan output and quantify the organization's strategic initiatives through volume, expense, and reimbursement projections that result in projected levels of net income, working capital, and cash reserves.

The system estimated its total cash flow available for capital spending in 2017 as approximately $31.1 million but then subtracted a 10 percent system capital contingency and a $500,000 preplanning contingency, yielding available net cash flow of approximately $27.5 million. Chapter 4 provides additional detail on contingency capital.

DEFENDING THE CONSTRAINT

After calculating the capital constraint, executives must ensure that organizational spending does not exceed this sum and that capital investment does not occur outside of the organization's capital allocation and management process. The capital management council must oversee the capital process at a high level. If the process breaks down and authorization of capital occurs outside the process, the validity of the capital constraint will be undermined and the integrity of the process diminished.

Leasing

In many organizations, the use of leasing is a significant challenge in determining the capital constraint. Some executives use, or try to use, operating leases to avoid including projects in the capital constraint calculation and the capital allocation and management process. Related issues include the following:

- Operating leases frequently represent the most expensive source of capital for an organization.
- Investment decisions must be independent both of executives' preferences and of financing decisions.

The second issue highlights an important corporate finance decision-making principle called the *separation theorem*. Applied to capital allocation and management, the principle states that investment decisions are best made by the

Exhibit 3.3 Calculating the Capital Constraint: Net Cash Available for Spending ($ in millions)

	2017	2018	2019	2020	2021
Operating income	$17,587	$12,950	$13,035	$14,104	$16,664
Nonoperating income (excluding interest)	6,364	9,864	7,989	8,064	11,039
Depreciation and amortization	25,167	29,226	33,335	36,677	39,309
Operating cash flow	49,118	52,040	54,359	58,845	67,012
New debt proceeds (net of restriction)	—	43,096	—	—	—
Non-income statement philanthropy	—	—	—	—	—
Interest income	4,885	4,583	4,820	5,431	6,177
Total sources of cash available for capital	54,003	99,719	59,179	64,276	73,189
Working capital requirements	(1,012)	(1,083)	(1,748)	(1,999)	(2,195)
Principal payments	(9,400)	(7,444)	(8,254)	(8,209)	(7,243)
Other sources or uses of cash	—	—	—	—	—
Carryforward capital	(23,104)	(12,949)	—	—	—
Contributions to cash reserves	(10,604)	(9)	(15,710)	(20,882)	(30,251)
Total uses of cash	(22,912)	(21,485)	(25,712)	(31,090)	(39,689)
Total cash flow available for capital spending	31,091	78,234	33,467	33,186	33,500
System capital contingency (10%)	(3,109)	(7,823)	(3,347)	(3,319)	(3,350)
Preplanning contingency	(500)	(500)	(500)	(500)	(500)
Net cash available for capital spending	$27,482	$69,911	$29,620	$29,367	$29,650
*Total capital spending**	$54,195	$91,183	$33,467	$33,186	$33,500

Add: Operating income ... Plus: New debt proceeds ... Less: Working capital requirements ... Less: Total cash flow available for capital spending

* Includes cash flow available for capital allocation and carryforward capital.

Source: Kaufman, Hall & Associates, LLC. Used with permission.

capital management council, and financing decisions are best made by the chief financial officer (CFO), who should have the broadest perspective of the organization's financial position and capital capacity. Department managers do not have this type of perspective.

Whether an organization considers a capital request within the capital constraint should be a function of the proposed investment's magnitude rather than the structure (i.e., financing) under which it will be acquired. Proposed expenditures (i.e., a lease for a medical office building, an outpatient facility, or a magnetic resonance imaging [MRI] machine) that meet the broad definition of threshold capital dollar levels should be subject to the capital constraint and included in the council's review and approval process.

Consider a health system that has established a capital constraint of $30 million, based on net income targeted in its financial plan, and has allocated the full $30 million. Two of the three high-end robots requested, totaling more than $5 million, did not make the cut. To appease the vocal department chair, or because an executive wanted the robots approved but was overruled by the council, the machines are leased after allocation of the capital constraint is completed.

The leases could create a zero footprint against the capital constraint (i.e., they could be solely an operating expense), but in this instance leasing has simply rationalized capital spending beyond the capital constraint. Spending is now $35 million rather than the established $30 million. In addition, because the capital constraint is a direct function of the organization's expected financial performance as projected in the financial plan, the higher spending level that leasing produces will negatively affect organizational cash flow beyond the current year. Total uses of cash throughout the lease period will be higher because of the lease-related payments, which are synonymous with debt service payments.

If the organization proceeds with the equipment leasing, its executives should consider why they established the $30 million capital constraint and why other capital-intensive projects should not be approved outside the established capital allocation and management process, given this violation of the spending limit.

The policy WHS established for the treatment of operating leases is designed to protect capital constraint integrity and maintain the transparency of review of high-dollar threshold requests within the established capital allocation and management process. In part, the policy states the following:

- Threshold capital items anticipated to be financed using an operating lease structure—whether new or renewal leases—will require review and approval by the capital management council or its designee.

- Capital expenditures financed through an operating lease will not affect the current-year threshold allocation of capital.
- Final approval of the use of operating lease financing will be contingent on the specific operating entity's continuing ability to meet its operating margin targets on a pro forma basis.

Healthcare debt-rating agencies closely assess an organization's use of operating leases to determine the effect of such financial obligations on the organization's debt capacity and credit quality. Since 2004, Moody's Investors Service has considered operating leases and other "innovative financing" techniques to be *on credit*. Therefore, in assessing debt capacity and credit quality, the agency has been incorporating leases as part of an organization's comprehensive debt program, "when material" (Moody's Investors Service 2004).

The Financial Accounting Standards Board officially changed the accounting treatment of operating leases in 2016, bringing all operating leases *on balance sheet*. The Financial Accounting Standards Board's February 2016 update to standards indicated that organizations that lease assets, whether through operating leases or capital leases, are required to recognize on their balance sheets the assets and liabilities created by leases with terms of more than 12 months. For public companies this provision will take effect after December 15, 2018; for all other organizations it will be effective one year later.

The new reporting standard treats operating leases as true, long-term financial obligations and requires organizations to identify leases' impact on the balance sheet, similar to the treatment of long-term debt. Consequently, the standard highlights the importance of reviewing, approving, and managing large operating leases through the capital allocation and management process.

Information Technology

Organizations should allocate capital for information technology (IT) the same way they allocate any other type of capital—within their capital allocation and management process. Doing so ensures comprehensive consideration of an IT project's short- and long-term benefits and costs within the organization's overall portfolio of investments.

Potential IT investments, like all potential major investments, should be included in the in-depth business planning and net-present-value analyses described in chapter 6. Analysis of IT capital should attempt to quantify, to the extent possible, all potential incremental operating costs and efficiencies over the life of the investment. IT initiatives likely will have a lower net present value than other projects in the organization's portfolio because of their infrastructure-like nature. However, like other infrastructure investments that represent basic costs of doing business, IT investments should be viewed within a balanced portfolio that is supported by objective analytics. If executives wish to proceed with the investment for qualitative rather than quantitative reasons, they will be fully aware of the investment's costs and likely financial implications.

An organization must clearly define how much capital it can afford to spend before it can define its capital pools, which is the subject of chapter 4.

New Era Calls on Cash

As described in this book's introduction and itemized in exhibit 1.1, the definition of capital has broadened to include everything that uses the organization's cash. Capital includes items such as a physician alignment strategy, business partnerships, and managed care products or plans. These items are large investments that will significantly affect the organization's liquidity and debt capacity, especially because measurement of that capacity is based on ongoing operating performance. Thus, organizations must include in their capital management process a broader definition of capital that captures these types of expenditures.

IMPLEMENTATION CONSIDERATIONS

An organization's capital constraint is a direct translation of its financial plan and a critical point of integration among its strategic, financial, and capital allocation processes. Without a sophisticated, multiyear financial plan, an organization will be unable to establish objective levels of capital spending for the upcoming year and to assess the impacts of its decisions on future years.

To determine the effectiveness of its financial plan, an organization should consider the following questions:

- Is the financial plan directly linked to the resource requirements and opportunities defined in the organization's strategic plan?
- Have specific credit goals related to profitability, liquidity, and capital structure been established?

- Does the financial plan simultaneously evaluate profit-and-loss projections and their related impacts on the balance sheet and cash flows of the organization?
- Have all sources and uses of cash been analyzed, including pension liabilities, working capital, risk-based reserve requirements, and others?
- Have operating and balance sheet risks and sensitivities been thoroughly quantified?

REFERENCES

Financial Accounting Standards Board. 2016. *Accounting Standards Update: Leases (Topic 842).* Norwalk, CT: Financial Accounting Standards Board.

Moody's Investors Service. 2016. *Outlook Stable as Cash Flow Growth Slows, But Remains Positive.* New York: Moody's Investors Service.

—. 2004. *Capital Access: Moody's View on Operating Leases: Off Balance Sheet But on Credit.* New York: Moody's Investors Service.

Wareham, T. 2015. "Addressing the Impact of New-Era Investments on Credit Ratings." Healthcare Financial Management Association *CFO Forum.* Published May 12. www.hfma.org/Content.aspx?id=30663.

CHAPTER 4

Defining the Capital Pools

THE NEXT STEP of a best-practice approach to capital allocation and management is to define the capital pools. By defining the capital pools, executives determine the portion of available dollars that will be centrally managed and allocated to capital investment opportunities that have been selected after rigorous analysis. Conversely, some of the available capital will be allocated to a pool for requests that do not warrant detailed business planning and analysis. The structural definitions in this chapter will help executives identify capital requests that require business planning analytics and will establish a means to manage the remaining requests that do not deserve such attention.

Healthcare organizations that have a well-designed capital allocation and management process define three investment pools—an approach recommended for all organizations:

1. Threshold capital pool
2. Nonthreshold capital pool
3. Contingency pool

The threshold and nonthreshold pools, described in more detail in the next section, should be the focus of allocation activity. The contingency pool, described later in this chapter, supports and provides reserves for investment activity that occurs through both the threshold and nonthreshold pools.

Why are there two pools for active allocation? Why not three or four, or just one? The capital allocation and management process is simply more efficient with fewer pools. Each pool has its own logistical, monitoring, and informational requirements, so fewer are better. Furthermore, the use of fewer pools minimizes organizational staff's ability to access funds for capital outside of the established process. Having only one big pool, however, creates an untenable management workload for executives who must then review all capital requests. This situation is likely to result in a lower standard of review for every request.

Many hospitals and health systems find the two-pool approach for active allocation generates positive results in terms of organizational acceptance, implementation, and financial performance. An organization's capital management council must clearly define the parameters for each pool and outline how capital in each pool should be accessed and managed. A discussion of these topics follows.

THRESHOLD AND NONTHRESHOLD CAPITAL

More than two decades ago, Kaufman, Hall & Associates introduced to healthcare the concept of threshold and nonthreshold capital. The concept stems from the best-practice corporate finance tenet: Capital requests that are at or above a specific dollar amount defined by an organization (i.e., the threshold) should benefit from comprehensive business planning analysis and centralized review. Expenditure requests referred to as *threshold capital* are equal to or more than the defined-dollar threshold amount, thus triggering analysis and review. *Nonthreshold capital* encompasses proposed capital expenditures that, on an individual basis, fall below the threshold dollar amount.

Setting the threshold is both an art and a science, but it should result in a definite number. The science involves analyzing historical requests and capital spending to determine the dollar level above which the vast majority—65 percent to 80 percent—of an organization's capital initiatives will require consistent, transparent, and rigorous quantitative analysis. The art is in evaluating how many project proposals are likely to be generated at a particular dollar threshold and assessing the organization's ability to appropriately prepare and review the required analyses.

An organization that manually analyzes capital projects may be able to manage only a small number of projects in support of the recommended one-batch review and allocation decision-making process each year, as described in chapter 2. On the other hand, an organization that uses a capital management software tool may be able to analyze and review as many as 40 or 50 projects as part of this annual process. Organizations that can prepare, review, and manage a large number of project analyses may consider setting a lower threshold dollar level, which ensures data-driven and high-quality decisions for a large proportion of planned capital spending.

Across healthcare, the defined dollar amount for threshold capital ranges from tens or hundreds of thousands of dollars at some small community hospitals to millions of dollars at large multistate and national health systems. Regardless of an organization's threshold dollar amount, the number should be hard and fast—in other words, it should be applied organization-wide without exception. Executives should review the capital threshold amount periodically (typically as a standard part of its annual capital allocation and management process) to ensure it remains appropriate.

Applying the capital threshold is straightforward. Any project with an associated multiyear total cost that is equal to or greater than the defined threshold dollar amount is considered a threshold capital project. Such projects should be funded from the threshold capital pool based on comparison with other proposed threshold capital initiatives, as described in chapter 6. This approach relies on a rigorous, standardized quantitative and qualitative analysis. Nonthreshold capital requests, on the other hand, are handled in a decentralized fashion, as described in chapter 5.

Establishment of a threshold and nonthreshold pool should not be confused with the creation of capital categories (often referred to as "buckets"). Defining capital investment categories (e.g., ambulatory capital, inpatient capital, routine capital) or capital investment types (e.g., IT capital, medical equipment capital, facility improvement capital) and allocating undifferentiated capital to them is neither advocated nor considered best practice. On the contrary, managing all capital comprehensively to reflect the organization's long-term strategic and financial vision is strongly recommended. Defining capital categories or types precludes thorough examination of whether those groupings are appropriate and warrant continued investment. It also disconnects the capital allocation and management process from the organization's strategic direction and from the evaluation of its overall portfolio value when making capital decisions. Exhibit 4.1 further describes traditional yet problematic approaches to capital pools.

FUNDING THE POOLS

In a best-practice capital allocation and management approach, organizations must define the principles under which net cash flow available for capital spending will be allocated among the three capital pools.

Allocation to the contingency pool is straightforward because it is typically a percentage of the organization's total cash flow available for spending. A review of capital management practices in health systems nationwide indicates that health systems' contingency pools typically vary between 5 percent and 15 percent, with the vast majority of systems allocating 10 percent of total cash flow to the contingency pool (Sussman 2016).

Funding levels for the threshold and nonthreshold capital pools are much more variable nationwide. However, the goal of a best-practice capital allocation and management approach is to ensure that the vast majority of an organization's capital spending—65 percent to 80 percent—undergoes rigorous analysis, as described earlier. This disciplined approach offers the added benefit of creating broader transparency and accountability around capital spending and the decision-making process.

Exhibit 4.2 illustrates how the two-hospital system described in chapter 3 (whose capital constraint calculation is illustrated in exhibit 3.3) apportions capital to the three pools. The system's total cash flow available for capital spending is $31.1 million. It allocates 10 percent of this amount, or $3.1 million, to the contingency pool and $500,000 to a preplanning contingency, leaving approximately $27.5 million as its net cash flow available for capital spending (i.e., its capital constraint).

Exhibit 4.2 Funding the Threshold and Nonthreshold Pools

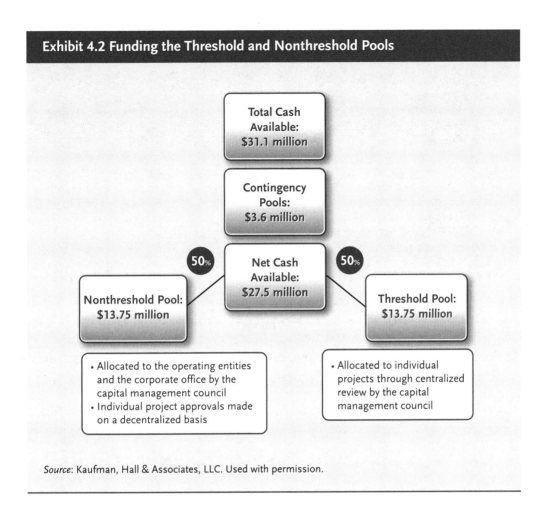

Total Cash Available: $31.1 million

Contingency Pools: $3.6 million

50%

Net Cash Available: $27.5 million

50%

Nonthreshold Pool: $13.75 million

Threshold Pool: $13.75 million

- Allocated to the operating entities and the corporate office by the capital management council
- Individual project approvals made on a decentralized basis

- Allocated to individual projects through centralized review by the capital management council

Source: Kaufman, Hall & Associates, LLC. Used with permission.

Because of significant levels of carryforward threshold capital in fiscal year 2017, the system allocates 50 percent of this sum to the threshold capital pool and 50 percent to the nonthreshold capital pool. Exhibit 4.3 illustrates how this results in approximately 72 percent of the annual capital expenditures being threshold in nature.

Many organizations apportion their defined capital constraint so that approximately 75 percent of it is to be spent as threshold capital under the capital management council's purview. Because the 75 percent includes carryforward capital, the actual apportioning of the current-year capital constraint between the threshold and nonthreshold pools may be 50:50; exhibit 4.3 illustrates the mathematics for such a situation.

The capital management council must evaluate the percentage allocations annually to account for changes in the amount of carryforward capital. The council should strive to oversee, through the centralized review and allocation process, approximately 75 percent of total capital spending. Any changes to the annual pool allocations should be made within the agreed-upon allocation structure.

Exhibit 4.3 Calculation of Total Allocation of Cash Available to Capital Pools

Net cash flow available for capital	$27,500
Add: Contingencies	3,600
Carryforward capital	23,100
Precommitted capital	—
Total allocated capital	**$54,200**
Net cash flow available allocated to	
Threshold capital at 50%	$14,000
Carryforward capital	23,100
Precommitted capital	—
50% of contingency capital	1,800
Total threshold capital	**$38,950**
Threshold capital as a percentage of total capital	**71.9%**

Source: Kaufman, Hall & Associates, LLC. Used with permission.

To do otherwise would create an unnecessary level of organizational uncertainty, potentially politicize the allocation process, diminish the process's transparency, and undermine the process's integrity.

MANAGING AND USING THE CAPITAL INVESTMENT POOLS

The capital management council governs the allocation and application of funds in an organization's three capital investment pools. Chapter 2 describes the structure, composition, and ongoing function of the capital management council, which should be defined by a documented policy.

Threshold Capital Pool

The threshold capital pool is the amount of money allocated to fund threshold capital requests, which are defined as capital projects whose total multiyear costs are equal to or exceed the preestablished dollar amount. Threshold capital projects have high-dollar costs and usually support the organization's strategic and financial plan.

The threshold capital pool should be managed centrally, under the aegis of a capital management council whose members represent key organizational constituencies. The council should govern all aspects of the threshold capital process to ensure the broadest context for decision making. In a healthcare system, threshold capital projects typically are system-based initiatives (e.g., electronic health record implementation). This fact further underscores the need for centralized evaluation and decision making. Chapter 6 discusses the evaluation of threshold capital initiatives in more detail.

Nonthreshold Capital Pool

Management of the nonthreshold capital pool should be decentralized. In a small stand-alone hospital, decisions regarding nonthreshold capital might be made at the vice president level. In a large academic medical center, decisions may be distributed according to scope of authority (e.g., clinical vs. administrative) and made by higher-level executives. In a multihospital environment, nonthreshold capital is usually managed at the local entity or regional level, where market-specific needs can be addressed.

Regardless of an organization's size and structure, the analytic requirements for nonthreshold capital will be far fewer than those for threshold capital. Most nonthreshold expenditures are ongoing in nature, such as those for low-dollar infrastructure and asset replacement needs.

Because each project drawing on the nonthreshold capital pool represents a small part of an organization's total capital spending, and because an organization typically has a large volume of low-dollar requests, an organization should collect information about nonthreshold capital requests using standardized categories and forms, as described further in chapter 5. Collecting information in this way is vital for efficient allocation and postallocation processes, including group purchasing decisions and the management of cash flow timing. Organizations can use capital management software to help gather and manage the necessary information.

Contingency Capital Pool

The contingency capital pool, which is deducted directly from the total cash flow available for capital spending before allocation of dollars to the other two pools, is intended to support threshold capital needs. The pool should be managed by the capital management council as a safety valve to fund the following items:

- Project cost overruns or operating performance shortfalls
- Unanticipated capital needs for emergencies (including code violations) that will materially affect a core business, patient safety, or the immediate quality of patient care
- Rare, off-cycle requests related to opportunities that truly were unknown at the time of the batch allocation process
- Preplanning costs related to determining initial cost estimates and scope of high-dollar, multiyear threshold projects, as described in chapter 3

The contingency capital pool should not be used to supplement the nonthreshold pool, which is managed on a decentralized basis. The capital management council also should determine how to handle unused contingency dollars. Should such dollars revert to the organization to supplement the following year's available dollars, or should they supplement current-year capital spending?

The answer to this question will vary by organization and by year. Nonetheless, the council should be vested with the authority to determine how unused contingency dollars are applied. The council can hold a broad, strategic discussion on this topic, leading to an enhanced decision. Often, unused contingency capital is divided between the threshold and nonthreshold pools using the same distribution methods that were employed initially.

CONCEPTS IN PRACTICE

Six-hospital academic health system Emory Healthcare, introduced in chapter 3, defines threshold capital projects as those requiring funding equal to or greater than $500,000. All new services and business ventures are considered to be threshold capital projects, to standardize and enhance business planning analysis, create transparency, and define accountability. Allocation of threshold capital is reviewed by the system's capital management council. Allocation of nonthreshold capital is reviewed on a decentralized basis by appropriate local management. In both cases, the review incorporates capital planning technology and key structural components similar to those used in the systemwide capital decision-making process, such as analytics, prioritization, and multidisciplinary governance.

Initially, Emory decided to allocate capital equally between the threshold and nonthreshold pools. In anticipation of its need to fund large, strategic initiatives, and as part of its multiyear process implementation plan, Emory will move to a 70 percent threshold and 30 percent nonthreshold allocation over the next few years. The systemwide council expects to review 40 to 60 threshold capital projects annually.

WHS, the four-hospital system described in chapter 3, defines threshold capital projects as those requiring funding equal to or greater than $350,000. Allocation of threshold capital is reviewed by the system's capital management council; allocation of nonthreshold capital is reviewed on a decentralized basis by operating executives of the appropriate entities, following review and prioritization by functional review committees. As at Emory Healthcare, all new business ventures at WHS are considered threshold capital projects.

WHS allocates 80 percent of its capital constraint to the threshold capital pool and 20 percent to the nonthreshold capital pool. These percentage allocations account for the level of carryforward threshold capital and precommitted capital going into the planning year. The systemwide council expects to review approximately 70 threshold capital projects per year.

Both Emory Healthcare and WHS allocate 10 percent of their total cash flow available for capital spending to a system contingency pool and an additional $500,000 for preplanning activities, as described in chapter 3.

After it has apportioned available capital into the threshold capital, nonthreshold capital, and contingency pools, an organization's capital management council can consider how to further allocate and evaluate nonthreshold capital, which is the subject of chapter 5.

IMPLEMENTATION CONSIDERATIONS

The concept of the threshold and nonthreshold capital pools is unique to capital management in several ways:

- The defined threshold level does not need to correlate to approval matrices, signature authorities, or other board governance–based policies and procedures.
- Through the increased transparency of the capital pool structure, the organization also has increased visibility into categories and types of capital to be spent prior to funding. As a result, in financial planning, capital investment business planning, and actual capital acquisition, an organization can better aggregate its portfolio information to assess the strategic alignment of its investment decisions, but also to take advantage of economies of scale and opportunities for negotiation.

- Many organizations choose to implement a higher threshold in the first year of a new capital allocation and management process to generate a more manageable threshold process workload. After gaining some experience with the process, an organization can manage and adjust the threshold to support its evolving needs.

REFERENCE

Sussman, J. H. 2016. *Survey of Capital Allocation Approaches in 26 U.S. Health Systems.* Skokie, IL: Kaufman, Hall & Associates, LLC.

CHAPTER 5

Allocating and Evaluating
Nonthreshold Capital

THIS CHAPTER DESCRIBES the recommended approach for allocating nonthreshold capital among the operating units that are developing appropriate uses for that capital. These operating units may include departments, service lines, regions, hospitals, ambulatory or post-acute facilities, physician clinics, and other organizational units.

Every operating unit has ongoing capital needs for replacing equipment (e.g., personal computers, patient monitors) and for infrastructure investments (e.g., lobby renovations, utility upgrades). Clearly, these requirements must be met for the unit to remain in operation and competitive. Meeting these requirements is a basic cost of doing business and therefore a long-term strategic requirement.

ALLOCATION PRINCIPLES

Basic capital cost notwithstanding, an organization's capital management council must make clear that funding for nonthreshold capital is not an annual right nor a gift that will automatically be given year after year. The organizational goal is to allocate nonthreshold dollars in a way that meets minimum capital needs and rewards performance at the operating-unit level. The allocation method should create incentives for each unit to contribute to organizational success by maximizing the dollars it receives.

Exhibit 5.1 lists principles for allocating nonthreshold capital that organizations can adapt to their specific needs.

An organization's approach to allocating nonthreshold capital to its operating units should address two key questions:

- Allocation of nonthreshold capital should be directed by the capital management council and driven formulaically based on each operating unit's performance relative to the organization's overall performance.
- The council always should retain the authority to adjust all formula-based allocations to ensure that every operating unit receives an appropriate minimum level of capital.
- All *provider units*, defined as units that generate patient revenue, must receive a minimum allocation of nonthreshold capital, as defined by the council, that is sufficient to meet the unit's basic needs (relative to its size, type of operation, and capital intensity).
- *Nonprovider units* should receive a minimum allocation of nonthreshold capital as determined by the council.
- The council should retain the authority to (1) adjust allocations based on unit-specific or market-specific considerations, and (2) reconsider the nonthreshold capital minimum annually and adjust it as appropriate.
- Once nonthreshold capital has been allocated by the council, units should manage it in a decentralized manner, using a capital decision-making process similar to the one used at the system level.

Source: Kaufman, Hall & Associates, LLC. Used with permission.

1. What measures should we use to link to unit and organizational long-term success the nonthreshold capital to be allocated to operating units?
2. How will we allocate nonthreshold capital to nonprofitable, non-revenue-producing, or small operating units?

The answers to these questions should prevent, or at least minimize, any gaming of the capital allocation and management process.

Allocation Measures

Health systems that have well-defined operating unit structures and continually measure unit-based performance can easily address the first of the two questions posed in the previous section. The best-practice allocation method currently used by US health systems is based on relative operating *earnings before interest, depreciation, and amortization expenses* (EBIDA). Used as a comparative measure, operating EBIDA assesses pure operating profitability and is not affected by a unit's past capital-related decisions.

For example, consider a unit that has underinvested in capital (i.e., not spent what it needs to spend to ensure market and financial performance as outlined in its strategic and financial plan). Because the underinvesting unit will have lower depreciation expenses than a unit that fully funds its capital needs, it will also have a higher operating margin (all other parameters being equal). If the organization allocates nonthreshold capital based on operating margin, the underinvesting unit will receive more capital than a unit that has been diligent about maintaining appropriate levels of capital investment. Thus, the underinvesting unit is rewarded for its behavior. In contrast, when the operating EBIDA method is used to allocate nonthreshold capital, the units are compared based on true, year-to-year profitability. Consequently, the underinvesting unit's behavior will not be rewarded, and the fully funded unit (assuming it has made wise capital investments) will receive more nonthreshold capital because of improved profitability through well-maintained and competitive facilities and equipment.

Applying the operating EBIDA method, the capital management council can evaluate individual units' historical operating performance and calculate each unit's relative contribution to overall organizational profitability. This contribution is best calculated as a percentage of total operating EBIDA over a defined period, typically at least 24 months and preferably 30 months. Using a period shorter than 24 months places the operating units at significant capital allocation risk based on the impact of a single bad year, which can result in a highly volatile allocation environment. Using a longer period—for example, 30 months—reduces such variability and rewards or withholds reward based solely on sustained trends. In addition, using a 30-month period allows the organization to include in the calculation the first 6 months of the current year as well as the two historical years.

The operating EBIDA approach also can be adopted by organizations that are not part of a multiunit system, but other approaches may be more effective for these types of organizations. Every organization has or should have internal performance measures that management employs to monitor success. Furthermore, most organizations have hierarchical management structures with delegated operating authority. For example, consider a community hospital that has the following management structure:

- Level 1 includes the CEO, chief operating officer (COO), chief financial officer (CFO), and other C-suite members.
- Level 2 includes vice presidents for different aspects of hospital operations (e.g., nursing, clinical services, support services, facilities).

How should this community hospital's capital management council allocate non-threshold capital to each vice president in an objective and consistent manner?

The council should keep two facts in mind:

1. Allocated nonthreshold dollars typically should be spent on low-dollar expenditures that have little (or no) expected financial return (i.e., they represent a basic cost of doing business).
2. Calculating operating EBIDA associated with each vice president's area of responsibility is difficult or impossible, especially for an executive such as the vice president of facilities, who has no revenue-generating departments under his or her purview.

For these reasons, the capital management council should define other performance measures. These measures will vary by organization; no one measure or combination of measures is correct for all organizations. Commonly applied measures for nonsystem organizations include the following:

- *Contribution to historical organization-wide operating and capital budget variances*: Low variances would be rewarded with more capital.
- *Number of full-time equivalents (FTEs), which would correlate people with capital*: Units with more people would receive more capital.
- *Relative percentage of operating costs*: Units with higher costs would receive more capital.

The first measure, which links low budget variances to higher capital, directly rewards vice presidents for appropriate cost management. The second measure, which links the number of staff to allocated capital, reflects the realities of hospital operations but could contribute to escalating costs resulting from "FTE creep." The third measure, which rewards departments with higher expenditures by giving them more capital, is neither desirable nor appropriate in a payment-constrained, cost-escalating environment moving to value-based payment.

Again, none of these methods is perfect, but an organization's council should give serious thought to adopting the most appropriate measure or combination of measures of specific performance.

Allocation to Non-Revenue-Producing, Nonprofitable, or Small Operating Units

How should nonthreshold capital be allocated to operating units that, because of their size, function, or historical financial performance, would receive an inadequate allocation of nonthreshold capital through a formula-based process?

Every health system or hospital has some operating units that fit this description. Each unit—whether a corporate office or several purely administrative departments—has capital requirements. An organization must have a reasonable mechanism for allocating nonthreshold capital to such units or operations to enable them to meet basic capital requirements.

Approaches to nonthreshold allocation vary by organization. One of the most popular approaches is to allocate a minimum dollar amount to all operating units. The challenge is to establish a minimum allocation in a manner that limits politics and maximizes objectivity. Most organizations that have successfully tackled this challenge have a broad-based governance structure, as described in chapter 2. By vesting this type of decision making in a capital management council rather than in the CEO or another individual, an organization typically can make a negotiated but objective minimum allocation of nonthreshold capital.

Small Health System Example

The capital management council of a two-hospital health system allocated 70 percent of its net cash flow available for capital to the threshold capital pool and 30 percent to the nonthreshold capital pool. The council determined that the hospital that contributed a bit more than 78 percent of the system's profitability during the past 30 months would receive a bit less than 78 percent of the system's nonthreshold capital allocation of 30 percent.

Exhibit 5.2 shows that the council allocated $50,000 to the corporate office even though the corporate office did not generate a positive EBIDA. The council established this minimum allocation in recognition of the corporate office's need to replace minor equipment. The council made funds available to support the $50,000 allocation by proportionately reducing the allocation to each of the two hospitals, effectively reducing Hospital A's allocation from 78.1 percent to 77.8 percent of nonthreshold capital.

Large Health System Example

The capital management council of an 11-hospital health system allocated its non-threshold capital using the operating EBIDA method. However, recognizing the

Exhibit 5.2 Allocating Nonthreshold Capital in a Two-Hospital Health System ($ in thousands)

	Profitability	% of Total Profitability	Allocated Nonthreshold Capital	Actual Percent Allocation
Hospital A	$ 83,834	78.1%	$11,207	77.8%
Hospital B	23,540	21.9	3,143	21.8
Corporate	0	0.0	50	0.4
Total system	$107,374	100.0%	$14,400	100.0%

Source: Kaufman, Hall & Associates, LLC. Used with permission.

insufficiency of the formula-based allocation for different units, the council also established a minimum level of nonthreshold capital for each unit. As indicated in exhibit 5.3, some of these levels were based on contractual obligations (e.g., Hospital G), while others reflected the fact that every unit needed some capital (e.g., the central business office and information systems).

The council established still other minimum levels based on its analysis of a unit's past spending levels and anticipated future needs. Using its established minimum allocations, the council adjusted allocation percentages to each of the operating units and defined specific dollar allocations.

When Allocated Nonthreshold Capital Is Considered Insufficient

An organization's capital management council should give an operating unit options to pursue if the unit believes its nonthreshold capital allocation is insufficient to fund its requirements. Providing options creates a "safety valve" to support needed capital spending that either would deplete allocated nonthreshold dollars or that represents a nonthreshold project that carries a competitive potential return on investment. The recommended approach provides two alternatives for the process design:

1. Individual capital requests that are greater than a defined amount (e.g., $100,000 or $500,000) may be moved to the threshold pool to compete for funding as part of the threshold capital review process. However, once a nonthreshold capital request is moved to the threshold capital process, control of its ultimate disposition must be passed from the unit's management to the capital management council. If a request has moved to the threshold capital

Exhibit 5.3 Allocating Nonthreshold Capital in a Large Health System ($ in thousands)

Unit	Operating EBIDA	Allocable Operating EBIDA	% of Total Operating EBIDA	Allocation of $13,608	Allocation Adjustments to Minimum	Allocation of $13,608	Final Allocation Percentage
Hospital A	$38,373	$38,373	38.3%	$5,206	$ —	$4,394	32.3%
Hospital B	29,839	29,839	29.8	4,049	—	3,417	25.1
Hospital C	13,530	13,530	13.5	1,836	—	1,549	11.4
Hospital D	5,060	5,060	5.0	687	—	579	4.3
Hospital E	340	340	0.3	46	125	125	0.9
Hospital F	905	905	0.9	123	125	125	0.9
Hospital G	3,118	3,118	3.1	423	750	750	5.5
Hospital H	845	845	0.8	115	370	370	2.7
Hospital I	—	—	0.0	—	—	—	0.0
Hospital J	8,286	8,286	8.3	1,124	—	949	7.0
Hospital K	—	—	0.0	—	—	—	0.0
Central business office	(45,549)	—	0.0	—	100	100	0.7
Laundry	—	—	0.0	—	100	100	0.7
Information systems	—	—	0.0	—	750	750	5.5
Corporate services	(45,549)	—	0.0	—	400	400	2.9
Education	—	—	0.0	—	—	—	0.0
Health centers	—	—	0.0	—	—	—	0.0
Total health system	$9,198	$100,296	100.0%	$13,608	$2,720	$13,608	100.0%

Source: Kaufman, Hall & Associates, LLC. Used with permission.

pool and the council does not approve it, the request should not be funded subsequently using nonthreshold dollars.
2. Additional dollars may be solicited directly from the capital management council. If these dollars are approved, the nonthreshold capital pool must be recalculated.

The rules that prohibit giving a unit control of nonthreshold capital after a request has been moved to the threshold pool or not approved for threshold funding are designed to eliminate the possibility of gaming the system. Methods of gaming the system include (1) submitting funding requests under both threshold and nonthreshold allocation approaches and (2) funding capital that is not approved in the threshold pool using allocated nonthreshold dollars.

EVALUATING NONTHRESHOLD CAPITAL PROJECTS

An organization must ensure that the evaluation and approval processes for non-threshold capital requests are as consistent as possible within the context of its decentralized management. The dollar amounts and impacts of nonthreshold capital requests are smaller than those of threshold capital requests. As a result, analysis of nonthreshold capital requests generally is not as comprehensive as that for threshold capital requests (for which development of complete business plans is recommended), but they should, in fact, be just as rigorous.

Because of the volume of nonthreshold capital requests, organizations should establish a rigid, defined structure to elicit information required for analysis. Organizations can streamline the submission, review, and sign-off processes by using planning software that provides templates for such requests. Using standard-ized capital request forms also ensures that required general information (e.g., item description, number of units, vendor, cost) is gathered. This information enables the organization to define and obtain other relevant information related to an investment's operating or financial benefits. Finally, having standardized data about a large number of requests helps the organization's supply chain function (i.e., pur-chasing) identify potential cost savings through volume purchasing or opportunities to standardize products.

Although an organization's capital management council does not need to review and approve specific nonthreshold requests, the appropriate departmental or orga-nizational body must evaluate them. For example, an organization benefits when all information technology (IT) nonthreshold requests undergo a functional review by a centralized IT team that focuses on the following criteria:

- Relevance of the request
- Consistency of the request with organizational standards and requirements
- Appropriateness of estimated costs and timing
- Opportunities for combining the request with other, similar requests to gain purchasing efficiency and other benefits

Similar functional-review committees could be established for nonthreshold capital requests for clinical equipment and minor facilities improvement. Through such reviews, operating unit management and the entire organization can achieve a consistent approach to specific types of nonthreshold capital investment.

Exhibit 5.4 shows a sample software-based form for identifying the rationale for nonthreshold capital requests, such as a request for bariatric beds. This organiza-tion's capital management council established specific financial and nonfinancial

Exhibit 5.4 Request Form for Nonthreshold Capital: Rationale

Bariatric Beds

Project Data

Project Type	Nursing	Project Type Detail	Bed
Department	26140 - EMC Emergency Room	Status	Approved

Project Details

Description	Bariatric beds for emergency department
Project Justification	There is a growing need for bariatric beds, and this is a patient safety enhancement.

Proposed Vendor	Company X	Purchase Period	April
Class	Strategic Plan	Reason	New Service
Category	Patient Care Equip/Pt Beds	Priority	Necessary for smooth operations

Capital-Related Questions

Capital Questions:	Response	Comments
Is purchasing review required for pricing?	Yes	
Is construction or renovation required?	Yes	Doors may need to be widened. Included $2,500 for renovation costs.
Does this project include an IT component?	No	
Is this request for medical equipment?	Yes	

Decision Matrix

Impact on Patient and/or Physician Satisfaction	Quality, Safety, & Compliance Effectiveness	Strategic & New Business Growth	Impact on Employee Work Experience
Modest positive impact for either	Substantial impact	Maintains our current business	Modest enhancement in dept only
Should bring us in line with industry standards/ trends.	This is a piece of equipment that provides much-needed safety for a population of our patients.	No new business expected.	Easier to care for larger patients.

Source: Kaufman, Hall & Associates, LLC. Used with permission.

criteria to be used in evaluating nonthreshold capital requests. These criteria are incorporated in the capital request form and its accompanying capital costs form (exhibit 5.5).

Many quantitative criteria that are applied to threshold capital (e.g., net present value, return efficiency, first-year positive cash flow, and internal rate of return) are not included on the nonthreshold capital form. Because of the nature of nonthreshold capital, operating impact assessment, showing incremental revenue and expenses, is another component of the nonthreshold capital request form. These quantitative items (not illustrated here) are estimated annually so that their effects can flow directly to the departmental operating budget if the capital is approved.

Exhibit 5.4 incorporates nonfinancial criteria, including the anticipated impact on patient or physician satisfaction; quality, safety, and compliance effectiveness; strategic and new business growth; and impact on employee work experience. This type of data helps an organization categorize the intent of the spending and measure the potential nonfinancial value of the proposed use of capital relative to other requests.

Additional evaluation of the data enhances informed decision making. As projects are approved, an organization can use planning tools to aggregate committed and planned spending for budgetary purposes and to better evaluate actual and committed spending versus budgeted spending. Having information about financial impact also enables management to measure, through budget variance analysis, the ultimate success of a purchase or investment.

Exhibit 5.5 Request Form for Nonthreshold Capital: Capital Costs

Bariatric Beds

	2017	Comments
Unit Cost	$15,000	
# Items	3	
Subtotal:	$45,000	
Additional Capital Costs Input		
IT Costs	$ -	
Facilities/Construction Costs	$2,500	Renovation costs to widen doors to rooms for new bariatric beds.
Clinical Engineering Costs	$ -	
Subtotal Additional Capital Costs Input	$2,500	
Shipping / Handling	$ -	
Other	$550	
Total Capital Request:	$48,050	

Source: Kaufman, Hall & Associates, LLC. Used with permission.

Because nonthreshold capital review is decentralized, the method for evaluating these capital requests, as implemented by operating unit executives, will reflect the unit's unique culture and structure. Although review processes may vary from unit to unit, their effectiveness is directly related to their objectivity and consistency. Furthermore, through transparent communication of nonthreshold capital decisions and the underlying reasoning, an organization can educate its managers and continually improve its nonthreshold capital request and decision-making processes.

IMPLEMENTATION CONSIDERATIONS

Employing a decentralized approach to nonthreshold capital allocation is an important step in building support for a best-practice capital allocation and management process. Delegating authority typically results in improved efficiency, supporting decision making that is directly aligned with a unit or division's requirements.

However, a decentralized approach can be daunting to executives who have little or no formal training or experience in finance. Boards and senior leadership teams must therefore give executives and managers the necessary tools, structure, and training to effectively address capital allocation and management responsibilities.

CHAPTER 6

Evaluating Threshold Capital Investment Opportunities

IMAGINE PLAYING BASEBALL with no rules. Three strikes do not make an out, so the neighborhood bully remains at the plate, swinging away for hours. When he tires, whoever races to the plate first gets to hit next. Teams do not have a set number of players on the field, so Team A has 18 people positioned between center field and right field, and Team B has only one player covering the entire outfield. Which team will win this game? Is this game even worth playing? Without a level playing field, wouldn't one team quit in disgust?

ONE-BATCH REVIEW

Capital allocation is certainly not a game, but fairness in hospital and health system executive suites is just as important as it is on the baseball field.

To ensure equal opportunity for every initiative under consideration, an organization must have a formal, one-batch review process that consistently applies uniform evaluative criteria, thereby facilitating direct comparison of competing capital initiatives.

In a one-batch review process, all projects—regardless of whether they are likely to generate a positive return on investment (ROI)—are reviewed, and capital is allocated, once a year as a complete portfolio of initiatives. Each investment opportunity (e.g., new ambulatory clinic, physician practice, quality initiative, decision support system) is considered within the entire portfolio of potential investments, as described later in this chapter.

In one-batch review, analysis of projects with a negative ROI is just as important as (and in some cases more important than) analysis of projects with a positive ROI.

If an organization's capital management council wishes to proceed with a profitless investment for reasons other than financial return, the organization will be fully aware of the economic costs and the likely outcomes of the expenditure.

Because it supports a portfolio perspective of capital allocation, the one-batch review approach eases process management and gives an organization complete control over the amount and type of capital expenditures it pursues. Thus, the organization can ensure that proposed capital investments and strategic goals are aligned.

For the one-batch approach to be successful, however, an organization must be able to view proposed capital expenditures within its integrated strategic and financial planning process. Such expenditures include the large multiyear projects or initiatives that an organization has evaluated through multiphase planning, as described in chapter 2. In addition, an organization's capital allocation decisions must be made in a timely manner to incorporate approved projects into its current-year operating and capital budgets.

Organizations that have established an integrated process calendar, such as the one described in chapter 2, can easily institute one-batch review. The approach has been successful at healthcare organizations of all sizes, structures, and operating orientations.

Objections to the use of one-batch review of capital include the project sponsors' belief that they cannot complete the required analysis in the established time frame because "we didn't learn of this investment opportunity until the last minute" or "we have too many projects and not enough time."

Organizations that have a well-designed capital management process question the validity of these objections. Because capital allocation is performed annually, it is similar to the existing, cyclical capital process at most organizations. Unforeseen, last-minute opportunities are rare, especially for large, complex projects. When they do arise, the capital management process must provide a mechanism for their review (as described in chapter 7) while maintaining total spending within the capital constraint. Senior managers should be aware of all projects requiring significant dollar investments. A corporate finance–based capital management process forces project champions to plan more rigorously to ensure that their analysis is ready for submission at the appropriate time to be considered for allocation of available capital.

BUSINESS PLANS AND STANDARDIZED FORMATS OR TEMPLATES

To facilitate informed decision making, each threshold capital investment opportunity should have a thorough business plan. This plan should describe the business concept and its strategic and financial effects in significant detail, thereby providing the basic documentation and analysis necessary for a valid capital decision.

All threshold capital project analyses should be developed and submitted using a single, standardized planning template. Uniform submissions help ensure true comparability and give an organization's executives and managers shared knowledge and vision of the key drivers of strategic financial success.

Information Required of All Threshold Capital Initiatives

Whether a threshold capital initiative is detailed in a business plan or in a threshold capital project review and approval form, its critical components are the following:

- Description of the proposed capital initiative
  - Consistency with and enhancement of the organization's mission and core values
  - Alignment with the organization's strategic plan and initiatives
- Details supporting the level of investment required to start and complete the proposed initiative
  - Amount and timing of the required capital investment
  - Projection of initial and ongoing operating requirements
  - Utilization projections and related assumptions
  - Delineation of the potential customers to be served and the way those customers will be attracted
- Detailed quantitative analysis to identify potential ROI and key financial risks associated with the investment
  - Projected financial impact (five or ten years, or at least two years beyond full project operationalization)
  - Projected cash flow
  - Net present value and expected net present value (risk adjusted)
  - Feasibility studies for fundraising and other sources of capital, as appropriate
- Qualitative factors
  - Effect on organization's competitive position in the market
  - Impact on critical groups of stakeholders
  - Influence on quality, outcomes, and cost of patient care
- Identification of potential exit strategies and related performance measures

This business planning information integrates data from sources, including strategic plan outputs, operating estimates, and capital estimates, to generate a complete, risk-adjusted view of an initiative's ROI (see exhibit 6.1). Key areas of business risk relate to achieving projected volume levels, controlling project investment, achieving anticipated operating efficiencies, and managing productivity. Risk analysis, as described later in this chapter, focuses on the relative importance, the probability of occurrence, and the impact of risk on a project's potential financial return.

Financial projections are a standard requirement in all business plans. To maintain validity throughout the organization, the projection development process should be supported by a standardized tool that

- defines a structured projection format;
- incorporates globally applicable assumptions established at an organizational level;
- requires specific delineation of all key assumptions;
- includes all quantitative and qualitative review criteria; and
- applies corporate finance–based techniques, such as weighted average cost of capital, discounted cash flow, and net present value.

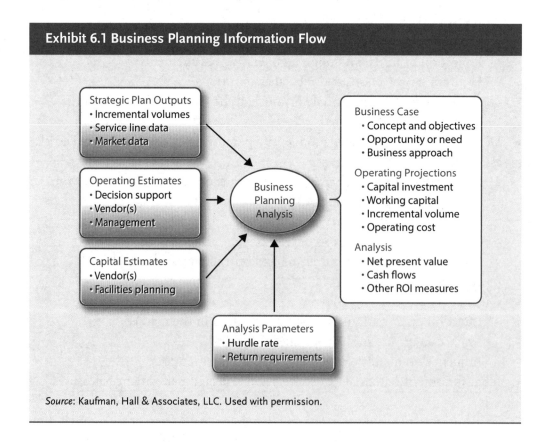

Exhibit 6.1 Business Planning Information Flow

Source: Kaufman, Hall & Associates, LLC. Used with permission.

The *quantitative* components of business planning for threshold capital opportunities focus on margin; the *qualitative* components focus on mission. Margin and mission can be balanced by weighting quantitative and qualitative factors during the decision-making process. This concept will be described in more detail later in this chapter.

QUANTITATIVE ANALYSIS USING CORPORATE FINANCE–BASED TECHNIQUES

Quantitative analysis using corporate finance–based techniques provides the fact base for informed decision making about capital investment opportunities. Organizations should work with key stakeholders to establish standardized evaluation and selection criteria for such opportunities for use to rank and score capital requests.

Most organizations include financial return as a significant project decision-making criterion, but seldom is it relied on as the only one. Furthermore, the weighting of financial return as a criterion varies among organizations. Organizations clearly cannot carry a series of investment decisions that do not add value to the organization. Best-practice capital management allows management discretion but applies rigorous analysis to ensure a transparent financial context for all decisions.

To effectively allocate capital, an organization must use the quantitative techniques typically used in corporate finance, such as the calculation of net cash flow available for capital, incremental cash flow projections, discounted cash flows, and net present value. In addition, assessing risk through techniques such as Monte Carlo simulation can be considered as another standard method to evaluate potential cash flows.

A consensus-driven approach to allocating capital that focuses solely on qualitative criteria does not provide the quantitative measures necessary to evaluate financial return of a project or portfolio of projects. Therefore, for each project under consideration, rigorous quantitative analysis should be performed to ensure a common language and outcomes or end points that can be compared. When push comes to shove, an organization's long-term viability and value stem from its ability to generate a financial return. Each project's return needs to be quantified. A *portfolio-based* positive return gives the organization the ability to invest in the next portfolio of strategies.

Return-on-Investment Methodologies

Standard methods for quantifying ROI include net present value (NPV), internal rate of return (IRR), payback period, annual return on capital (ROC), and annual return on equity (ROE). These terms are defined in exhibit 6.2.

NPV, a core analytical approach used in corporate finance, distills a project's financial ebbs and flows to a single dollar value. IRR calculates the interest rate needed to generate an NPV of zero. Although these approaches mirror one another, they have a few significant differences. IRR assumes that all cash flows generated will be reinvested at the same interest rate (i.e., the IRR), which may not happen. In other words, cash flows generated by a project with an IRR of 15 percent are assumed to earn 15 percent interest. This assumption may be overly optimistic. Moreover, it is difficult, if not impossible, to use IRR to evaluate a project that has no up-front capital investment.

For example, consider an initiative to develop a new service or program. The required initial investment would be limited to new staff and operating supplies for the first six to nine months of operations. The investment costs would not be depre-

---

Exhibit 6.2 Return-on-Investment Methodologies

Net present value (NPV)

A project's net contribution to financial performance—the value of future cash flows in today's dollars minus the required initial investment

Internal rate of return (IRR)

The rate of interest that discounts future net inflows from the proposed investment down to the amount invested (i.e., the rate of discount that makes NPV = 0)

Payback period

The length of time required for cash generated from an investment to equal the amount of cash originally invested in the project

Annual return on capital (ROC)

The annual net income generated by a project investment as a percentage of the original total project investment

Annual return on equity (ROE)

The annual net income generated by a project investment as a percentage of the original equity invested in the project

---

ciable; rather, they would be incremental operating costs associated with the new service. Without a definable capital cost, IRR analysis fails. In contrast, such a project would be easily evaluated using NPV, which tracks cash inflows and cash outflows, distinguishing cash flows only by their timing and not by their underlying nature.

Payback period looks at the sequence of cash flows out and in to determine the point at which they each equal one another. ROC evaluates the annual net income generated by a project relative to the total amount of capital invested in the project. If an organization invests $1 million to purchase a piece of equipment that generates net income of $200,000, the ROC is 20 percent. ROE evaluates the net income generated by a project relative to the total amount of original equity invested in the project. For example, if the same $1 million equipment purchase is financed by an $800,000 capital lease, the equity investment is only $200,000. If the equipment generates net income of $200,000, the ROE is 100 percent. ROE is commonly used to evaluate real-estate development and leasing investments. Another term for ROE is *cash-on-cash return*.

Although each of these methods can contribute positively to comprehensive project analysis, the degree to which each method accounts for the following important factors varies (see exhibit 6.3):

- *Noncapital investment*: Cash investment needed to initiate a project; it is used for purposes other than land, facilities, or equipment.
- *The time value of money*: A dollar today is worth more than a dollar in the future.
- *Project return over its lifetime*: The timing and magnitude of cash flows generated by investments vary by project.
- *Financing assumptions*: Assumptions include whether the investment is financed through debt, leasing, or another external financing mechanism.

Exhibit 6.3 Comparison of ROI Methodologies

Method	Accounts for Noncapital Investment?	Accounts for Time Value of Money?	Accounts for Project Life Return?	Includes Financing Assumptions?
NPV	Yes	Yes	Yes	No
IRR	No	Yes	Yes	No
Payback period	Yes	No	Yes	Yes
ROC	Yes	No	No	Yes
ROE	Yes	No	No	Yes

Source: Kaufman, Hall & Associates, LLC. Used with permission.

The aforementioned ROI methodologies, except for IRR, take into account noncapital investment. Only NPV and IRR account for the time value of money, working backward over the life of a project to evaluate the value (and opportunity costs) in today's dollars.

NPV, IRR, and payback period evaluate ROI over the life of a project. ROC and ROE are annual measures and therefore do not consider an investment's return over the project's life or the time value of money. Payback period, ROC, and ROE include interest cost in net income calculations.

Financing assumptions, such as interest cost in a "lease versus buy" decision, should be separated from the actual investment analysis. Only NPV and IRR properly separate investment and financing decision making. Investment decisions should focus on the appropriateness and potential value of a project; financing decisions for selected projects should be made on a portfolio basis at the corporate treasury level.

Applying all five methodologies concurrently typically provides a complete picture of a project's ROI, but even the most sophisticated organizations are unlikely to do this because of the time and effort involved. Instead, many healthcare organizations choose to use the NPV and IRR methods for project analysis. These organizations identify a hurdle rate (i.e., the required rate of return; sometimes referred to as the "discount rate") that the portfolio of investment opportunities should generate to meet the cash flow requirements of the organization's long-term capital plan.

Many organizations calculate the payback period for projects with a positive NPV. The payback period defines how long it will take to recover invested cash and at which stage in the project's life the NPV is generated. If a project with a positive NPV has a long payback period, the organization knows it will need to rely on longer-term cash flows to generate the positive return.

Expected-net-present-value (ENPV) analysis, which adds risk to the NPV analysis, is the most valuable technique for analyzing a potential investment. Because ENPV analysis builds on NPV analysis, one must thoroughly understand the components of the NPV method before applying risk assessment approaches.

Net-Present-Value Analysis

As mentioned earlier, NPV analysis is a straightforward, reliable technique that distills the financial ebbs and flows of a project to a single dollar value. NPV analysis enables a project to be evaluated on its own merits and helps explain how the project compares financially to others under consideration. Generally, a project requires some initial investment. The investment is followed by a start-up period during which financial (i.e., cash flow) losses may occur. Then, hopefully, net cash flows from the project approach zero and the project enters a period of financial performance that represents actual financial gain (i.e., positive cash flows).

NPV is based on two principles: (1) a dollar today is worth more than a dollar in the future, and (2) higher risks require higher rewards. NPV analysis compares the present value of the amount and timing of cash inflows of different projects to the present value of the amount and timing of their cash outflows, applying a consistent hurdle rate to represent the organization's ROI requirement over time. The calculation of NPV is shown in exhibit 6.4.

A project with a positive NPV represents an investment whose return is greater than the organization's financial hurdle. The investment's inflows are greater than its outflows, when all such flows are viewed in today's dollars and a specified interest rate is assumed. In comparing two or more projects, the higher a project's NPV, the more attractive it is from a strictly financial perspective.

Four elements must be known to perform valid NPV analysis: (1) an estimate of the amount and timing of up-front investment requirements, (2) the projection of free cash flows, (3) the organizational hurdle rate, and (4) the terminal value of the project.

Up-Front Investment Requirements

If a proper business plan has been developed for a project, the estimated amount and timing of the up-front investment needed for the project should be reasonably clear. Only incremental investment should be included, ignoring outlays already made even if they are project related. These prior investments are, in effect, sunk costs (i.e., costs already incurred that remain unchanged regardless of any future decision related to the project).

While focusing on incremental costs, organizations should be sure to include opportunity cost as part of the required project investment. *Opportunity cost* is defined as the difference between (1) the benefits earned through investment in one use of capital and (2) the yield that capital could have earned, such as interest earnings, had it been placed in an alternative investment generating the highest-possible yield. For example, a project proposal to construct a building on land that otherwise could be sold for a certain price should include the gain from the sale value of the land as an opportunity cost.

Requirements for working capital should be a final consideration in developing an estimate of total up-front project investment. Initial funding requirements, such as start-up operating expense subsidies or support required until accounts receivable are collected, must be paid from cash reserves until the project generates sufficient cash flow to carry these costs on its own.

Exhibit 6.4 Calculating Net Present Value

The future value of a present sum of money is expressed as $FV = PV (1 + r)^t$ where:

$$FV = \text{Future value}$$
$$PV = \text{Present value}$$
$$r = \text{Interest rate}$$
$$t = \text{Number of time periods}$$

By rearranging the above terms, it is possible to express the present value of a future cash flow as follows:

$$PV = \frac{FV}{(1 + r)^t}$$

The present value of an investment decision that results in a series of future cash flows may be expressed as follows:

$$NPV = C_0 + \frac{C_1}{(1 + r)^t} + \frac{C_2}{(1 + r)^2} + \frac{C_n}{(1 + r)^n}$$

where

$$NPV = \text{Net present value}$$
$$C_0 = \text{Up-front expenditure associated with the investment}$$
$$C_0, C_2 \ldots C_n = \text{Particular cash flows expected in particular periods}$$
$$r = \text{Interest (or discount) rate}$$

As an example, assume that an investment of $50 now would yield cash flows of $25 per year for three years and that the discount rate is 10 percent. The NPV of that investment would be:

$$(\$50) + \frac{\$25}{1.1} + \frac{\$25}{(1.1)^2} + \frac{\$25}{(1.1)^3} = (\$50) + 23 + \$21 + \$19 = \$13$$

In corporate finance theory, the decision rule is that the investment is acceptable if it has a positive NPV, because this means that the investment generates more than the opportunity cost of capital.

Source: Kaufman (2006). Reprinted with permission.

Projection of Free Cash Flows

The projection of free cash flows involves determining how much cash will be generated in a particular year from the ongoing operation of the proposed project:

Projected free cash flow = Projected net income + Depreciation
– Projected increases in working capital requirements – Estimated capital expenditures

Appropriate free cash flow projections *exclude* the following three categories of expense that would otherwise appear on a projected income statement:

- *Depreciation*: Depreciation is a noncash expense.
- *Allocation of overhead*: Overhead is fixed and is not incurred as a result of the proposed project; it exists regardless of the proposed project. If, however, a project truly creates an incremental change to overhead costs, only that increment should be included as an expense in free cash flow projections.
- *Cost of capital (interest expense)*: The basic tenet of corporate finance mandates separation of investment decisions and financing decisions. Financing alternatives should be considered separately after a portfolio of projects has been identified, as described later in this chapter. Thus, projections of free cash flows should assume that the project investment is 100 percent equity. Interest and principal payments should not be included in the projections.

These three exclusions aside, organizations should remember to do the following:

- Explicitly estimate the incremental effects of factors such as increased market share or operating efficiencies attributable to the proposed investment.
- Incorporate the effects of inflation on revenues and expenses.
- Include any incremental ongoing capital requirements necessary to keep the project going.

Organizational Hurdle Rate

The organizational hurdle rate determines the value of future cash flows relative to investment of like dollars today in interest-earning vehicles. If a project is risky, it should have a higher expected return than a relatively risk-free investment. Organizations should consider questions such as, How should an appropriate hurdle rate be established? How should the discounted cash flow analysis account for the relative risk of an investment?

The answers to these questions vary among both nonhealthcare and healthcare organizations. Many methods are used to calculate the organizational hurdle rate, but all conclude that the real cost of capital to an organization is significantly higher than simply its cost of debt. Some organizations apply a rule of thumb that sets the hurdle rate at two times the risk-free rate (i.e., the interest rate on 30-year Treasury bonds). Thus, if the current Treasury rate is 2.35 percent, the applicable hurdle rate would be 4.70 percent. This approach, however, provides limited accountability for the organization's return on invested equity.

Although rules of thumb may be straightforward and easy to apply, they are not the best approach to setting an appropriate hurdle rate. To quickly test the validity of an established hurdle rate, organizations should divide their current operating EBIDA margin (operating earnings before interest, depreciation, and amortization expenses) by total operating revenue. This ratio indicates the free cash flow return being generated by the organization's current operations and establishes a floor for future capital investments. If current operations are generating a certain percentage cash return, why should the organization settle for anything less from future invested capital?

The financial community uses the *weighted average cost of capital* (WACC) as the most appropriate measure of the required return on a project investment. This measure incorporates both a necessary return on debt-supported capital and a return on invested equity. Even though not-for-profit organizations do not issue stock (equity) or pay out dividends to shareholders, they still need to generate sufficient capital to ensure ongoing reinvestment in growth and mission. Thus, the hurdle rate should reflect the organization's WACC, which, by including an equity return element, ensures generation of reinvestment capital.

The WACC is defined as the percentage of debt multiplied by the organization's cost of debt capital, plus the percentage of equity multiplied by the organization's equity cost of capital. The WACC thus incorporates both the cost of equity and the cost of debt. It should be recalculated at least annually. Exhibit 6.5 illustrates how to calculate the WACC.

Terminal Value of a Project

The terminal value of a project is the investment's estimated value at the end of its operational life (i.e., the point at which significant additional capital investment will be required for the project to continue to generate cash flow). Terminal value can account for 30 percent to 60 percent of an investment's total value; therefore, it must be estimated carefully and documented thoroughly.

Terminal value can be estimated in four ways:

1. Assume *no value*, which would be appropriate for an item such as a computer that has no material value at the end of the project's life.
2. Calculate *liquidation value*, based on the assumption that the asset has an anticipated sale value at the end of the project's life.
3. Calculate an *annuity value*, which assumes that the investment will continue to generate free cash flow equal to that of the last projected year of the proposed project's life, during a period ranging from one year past the project's last year to a perpetuity.
4. Calculate a *growth annuity value*, which is similar to the basic annuity value, but assumes that the level of free cash flow after the projection period will change annually.

The terminal value of a project accrues at the end of the project's life. To define the true benefit of terminal value, the projected future value must be discounted back to today (i.e., the beginning of the project's life) using the hurdle rate applied to all other cash flows.

Other Issues Related to Net-Present-Value Analysis

Other issues associated with NPV analysis of proposed project investments include identifying the project's life and cash flow timing. Many organizations struggle with the following questions: What is the appropriate life for the project? Considering the pace of change in healthcare and the breadth of unknown factors, is it possible to develop an analysis for a 10- or 30-year project that is credible?

With NPV analysis, the project's life is not equal to the asset's depreciable life. For example, the depreciable life of a computed tomography (CT) scanner may be seven years for accounting purposes. If an organization routinely operates such equipment for ten years, however, it can establish the scanner's life for NPV purposes as ten years. If that is the case, the organization should include increasing maintenance costs, downtime, and clinical obsolescence in the latter years of the cash flow projections. In this example, free cash flow will probably peak around the fifth year and then decline, perhaps rapidly, during the subsequent years. Because the smaller cash flows in the latter years are discounted back to the present through the NPV analysis, the incremental impact of the CT scanner's extended life is likely to be minimal. An organization could review its equipment use history to help establish appropriate project life spans.

The issue of project life is especially significant for multiyear construction projects. Because any incremental cash flows generated by the investment will not begin for several years, a short project life will invariably generate a negative NPV. On the other hand, assigning a 30-year project life, which would support a positive NPV, may create an unrealistically long period for achieving ROI. One approach to addressing this issue is simply adding a fixed number of years (e.g., 15) to the project investment period to create a finite project life. In this way, even for a project with an extended construction period, the NPV analysis provides for a sufficiently long operating period in which to evaluate net cash flows.

An organization should also consider expected cash flows and their timing. When large projects are layered on top of one another, cash flow becomes critical. Multiple projects that all have negative cash flows in their early years can sink an organization. For this reason, an organization should combine its NPV analysis with an evaluation of the proposed project's cash flow implications.

Considering Risk Through Expected-Net-Present-Value Analysis

The projections supporting NPV analysis are based on a set of planning assumptions that include incremental volume, revenue, expense, cost and revenue inflation, and required capital, all of which may or may not be accurate. If the assumptions are optimistic and overestimate the project's financial return, the organization may be at considerable risk for overinvesting relative to its financial capability (i.e., spending more capital than it can afford).

To strengthen NPV analysis, organizations can use risk assessment techniques to integrate quantification of project risk into the investment return calculation. For example, Monte Carlo simulation bombards projections for an individual project or a portfolio of projects with a range of assumptions associated with key risk elements and generates a distribution of possible outcomes. Using simulation to further analyze projects generates a better estimate of the range of potential outcomes and, therefore, the risk-adjusted value of projects under consideration. This risk-adjusted return is the ENPV.

Suppose a hospital is considering investing in a new diagnostic imaging modality. The project's NPV is estimated to be $585,882, based on the specified assumptions of incremental demand and operating costs driving the projections of cash flow (see exhibit 6.6). This NPV point estimate is not necessarily the project's risk-adjusted ENPV. Simulation will provide a range of NPV outcomes, applying randomly generated combinations of demand and operating assumptions, to create the ENPV. The ENPV indicates the investment's likely return, incorporating risk, and illuminates potentially hidden risks, even for a project with a high NPV.

Use of simulation with this example indicates that the diagnostic imaging modality could have an NPV ranging from more than positive $500,000 to as low as negative $600,000. Exhibit 6.7 shows that the ENPV (the mean NPV of the range of possible outcomes) for the project is $122,000. The project thus has a positive return even when all potential risks and their impact on the range of assumptions generating the free cash flow projections are considered. However, the simulation also indicates that the probability of generating the $585,882 point estimate projected in the standard NPV analysis is far less than 100 percent. The hospital can better compare this initiative with other initiatives under consideration using the risk-sensitized ENPV.

Another view of the range of possible outcomes provides even better insight into this proposed investment's potential return and risks. Exhibit 6.8 essentially is exhibit 6.7 turned on its side to present the cumulative effect of all the calculated individual NPV probabilities. The chart indicates that there is an approximately 38 percent probability that the proposed diagnostic imaging investment will generate a negative NPV, and an almost 100 percent probability that the project will generate cash flows less than the point estimate projection. In other words, when risk is included in the analysis, there is little chance of achieving the NPV of $585,000.

Risk adjustment, also known as *sensitivity analysis*, should be consistently applied to all threshold capital projects. However, an organization should customize

Exhibit 6.6 Net Present Value Computation

Projected Free Cash Flow Analysis

	2017	2018	2019	2020	2021	2022	2023
Income from operation	$0	$0	($51,811)	($178,923)	$271,149	$489,727	$743,512
Add back: Depreciation and amortization	0	0	188,214	365,786	371,143	376,500	381,857
Less: Ongoing capital needs	0	0	0	75,000	0	75,000	0
Working capital	0	0	36,815	12,656	62,570	35,169	40,778
Net free cash flow	$0	$0	$91,589	$99,207	$579,722	$756,057	$1,084,591

Net Present Value Computation

Year	Capital Investment	Initial Cash Flows	Project Cash Flows	Total Terminal Value	Discounted Cash Flow	Cumulative Discounted Cash Flow
2017	$0	$0	$0		$0	$0
2018	(2,025,000)	0	(2,025,000)		(2,025,000)	(2,025,000)
2019	(750,000)	91,589	(658,411)		(597,096)	(2,622,096)
2020	0	99,207	99,207		70,803	(2,551,294)
2021	0	579,722	579,722		369,743	(2,181,551)
2022	0	756,057	756,057		430,927	(1,750,623)
2023	0	1,084,591	1,084,591		552,441	(1,198,183)
Terminal year				3,919,414	1,784,064	585,882
Total	($2,775,000)	$2,611,166	($163,834)	$3,919,414	$585,882	

Perpetuity cash flow change	0.0%
Total project life (in years)	10 years
Net present value of net free cash flow at 11.9%	$585,882

Source: Kaufman, Hall & Associates, LLC. Used with permission.

the analysis to reflect the specific risk parameters applicable to the project-related assumptions.

For example, one organization established a policy to assess the potential risk associated with each threshold capital project by estimating high and low assumption ranges for the following categories, as appropriate:

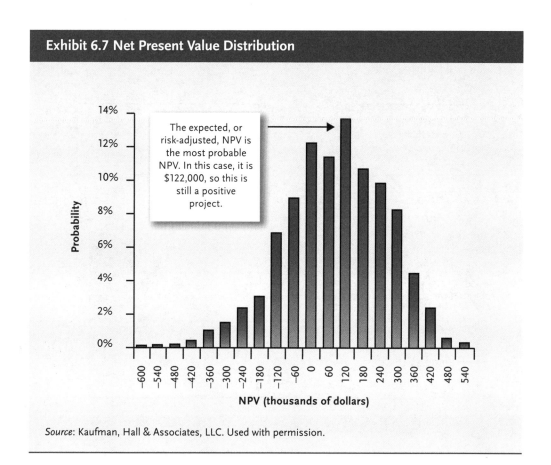

Exhibit 6.7 Net Present Value Distribution

The expected, or risk-adjusted, NPV is the most probable NPV. In this case, it is $122,000, so this is still a positive project.

NPV (thousands of dollars)

Probability

Source: Kaufman, Hall & Associates, LLC. Used with permission.

- Incremental project-related volume
- Incremental project-related revenue
- Reimbursement inflation by payer type
- Beginning salary levels by full-time equivalent (FTE) type
- Annual salary inflation levels
- Annual variable-expense inflation levels
- Annual fixed-expense inflation levels
- Initial capital investment requirements
- Increase or decrease in annual-perpetuity cash flow levels

The upside and downside scenarios generated by sensitivity analysis can be significant. Using Monte Carlo simulation, exhibit 6.9 (a tornado graph) focuses on how the identified risk components drive the projected ENPV of the diagnostic imaging modality investment example.

This tornado graph provides information that is valuable to both the project's sponsor and the organization's capital allocation decision makers. The project's highest risk is associated with changes in future reimbursement inflation. The

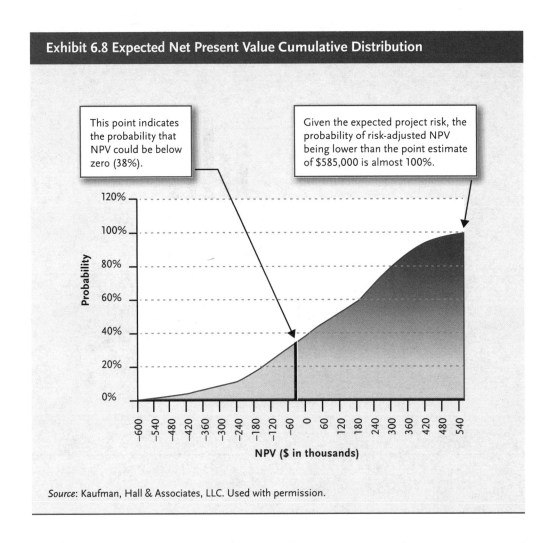

Exhibit 6.8 Expected Net Present Value Cumulative Distribution

This point indicates the probability that NPV could be below zero (38%).

Given the expected project risk, the probability of risk-adjusted NPV being lower than the point estimate of $585,000 is almost 100%.

Probability

120%

100%

80%

60%

40%

20%

0%

−600 −540 −480 −420 −360 −300 −240 −180 −120 −60 0 60 120 180 240 300 360 420 480 540

NPV ($ in thousands)

Source: Kaufman, Hall & Associates, LLC. Used with permission.

reimbursement inflation bar's extension to the right of zero indicates a positive and direct correlation between higher inflation (i.e., higher net revenue) and higher project NPV. In addition, the graph highlights the significant negative correlation between capital investment and NPV. This relationship may seem obvious, but in many organizations capital investment is one of the least challenged assumptions, even though reduction in capital investment requirements has a dollar-for-dollar positive impact on project NPV.

The positive correlation between discharges and NPV, as opposed to the lack of correlation between procedural volumes and NPV, indicates that the ancillary service provision, as structured in the proposal, is not profitable. The project relies on inpatient referrals to generate cash flow.

Through the tornado graph, management can see that it needs to carefully assess the diagnostic imaging modality investment's proposed operating structure to determine if changes can be made to enhance cash flows, mitigate project risk, and maximize potential project return. This assessment is especially needed considering healthcare's transition from volume-based payment to a more episodic, value-based structure. Generating more volume may be a benefit in the short run, but the analysis also must consider the impact of a fundamental change in payment structure. This proposed investment derives its positive return from the current structure of reimbursement; should that change, as is possible given current trends, the ENPV analysis shows that the investment's success would be at significant risk.

The increase in large capital projects in healthcare (e.g., physician practice acquisitions or integration, new nonacute care businesses with multiyear up-front investments and limited short-term returns) has highlighted the need for increased analysis of project risk and comparison of the risks of multiple projects. The traditional approach of creating optimistic, pessimistic, and expected scenarios is no longer

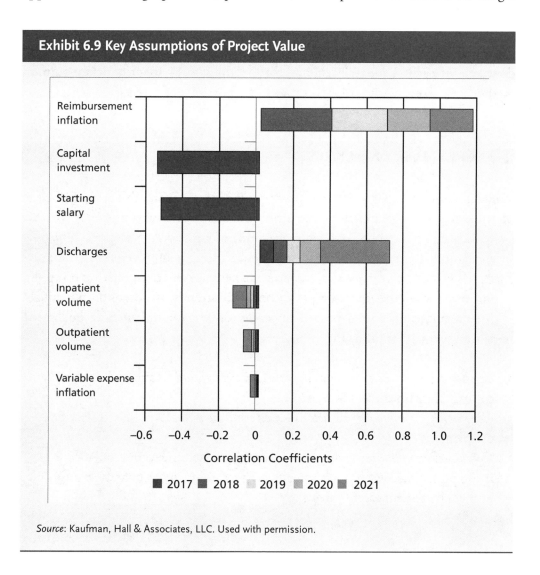

Exhibit 6.9 Key Assumptions of Project Value

Source: Kaufman, Hall & Associates, LLC. Used with permission.

sufficient to explain potential risk factors and their quantifiable effects. To support the evaluation of alternative investments being considered for a comprehensive capital portfolio, organizations must address questions such as the following:

- How are project risk factors identified?
- What are the best approaches to quantifying risk for different project types?
- Should risk be evaluated on a project-specific basis or with broad risk factors?
- Should target rates of return be changed to reflect risk?
- Should project risk be assessed by an entity or department, or by the overall organization?

To decide which investments to pursue, healthcare leaders must assess each project's risk parameters by using ENPV as the ROI method of choice. Because of the pace of market- and reform-related change in healthcare, hospitals and health systems should use scenario and sensitivity analyses to understand the upside and downside of each element in exhibit 6.10. Exhibit 6.11 identifies the common methods for assessing the risk of a project or a portfolio of projects.

QUALITATIVE ANALYSIS

While quantitative analysis focuses on financial return, qualitative analysis focuses on issues that are more difficult to quantify, including mission; consistency with the strategic plan; community needs; and effect on patient and staff safety, quality, physician alignment, innovation, customer value, and process improvement. Qualitative analysis is subjective; it reflects each analyst's experience and perspective at one point in time, even when the analysis is performed concurrently by dozens of individuals.

An organization's initial project-screening criteria should include qualitative measures, such as the following:

- *Consistency with the organization's mission, vision, and values*: Is the project compatible with these domains?
- *Consistency with the organization's stated strategic plan*: Does the project fit the plan?
- *Regulatory compliance*: Is the project compliant with relevant regulations? Is the project needed to meet a regulatory requirement or to address an immediate patient safety threat?

Exhibit 6.10 Scenario and Sensitivity Checklist for Reform-Related Change

Scenario and sensitivity analyses of the following factors can help hospitals and healthcare systems better gauge the impact of the changing healthcare delivery and payment landscape on investment opportunities:

- **Volume trends:** Inpatient admissions, outpatient clinic or physician office visits, emergency department visits
- **Payment rates:** Medicare (disproportionate share payments, penalties), Medicaid, and commercial insurers
- **Payer mix:** Commercial, Medicare, and Medicaid
- **Narrow network participation:** Inclusion or exclusion
- **Market share increases or decreases:** Geographic, or covered lives under population health models
- **Expenses:** Operating and nonoperating
- **Bad debt and uncompensated care:** Increases or decreases

Source: Kaufman, Hall & Associates, LLC. Used with permission.

Exhibit 6.11 Methods to Assess the Risk of Capital Projects

The most common risk-assessment techniques include the following:

- **Two-dimensional impact or probability:** Assesses a risk's relative impact and likelihood of occurrence based on qualitative information
- **Sensitivity analysis:** Evaluates what will happen if key assumptions change and identifies the range of change within which the project will remain profitable; can be used to determine which variables have the greatest influence on risk, as described earlier
- **Decision-tree analysis:** Graphically outlines potential scenarios and calculates each scenario's expected profitability based on the project's cash flow and net income
- **Monte Carlo simulation:** Uses econometric and statistical probability analyses to find the uncertainties of some *dependent* variables based on the assumed uncertainties of a set of *independent* variables; used to determine whether the total risk of a project is too great to allow it to proceed
- **Economic value added:** Adjusts income for accounting distortions that decrease short-term income but have long-term effects on future economic value

Sources: Adapted from National Research Council (2005); Wilkinson (2013).

These questions require simple *yes* or *no* answers. *Yes* means that the project should be retained on the list of investment proposals; *no* means that the project should be demoted to the bottom of the list or even eliminated from consideration.

If these binary questions generate significant discussion, the organization's leaders may be trying to bend the initiative or the organization's stated mission, vision, values, and strategic plan to achieve a fit for a project that otherwise would be rejected. Members of the capital management council should be alert to this situation and ensure that the allocation decision makers maintain a corporate perspective rather than a project-champion perspective.

If the project is needed to meet a regulatory requirement or to address an immediate patient safety threat, leaders should move the project to the top of the list of investment proposals and approve it. The dollars associated with this approval should be deducted from the organization's cash flow available to fund capital (i.e., its capital constraint).

Additional qualitative criteria vary among organizations. Executives should identify and agree on the criteria that will be used to evaluate potential initiatives; all proposed projects should be evaluated based on these criteria.

Exhibit 6.12 provides an example of the qualitative criteria and related questions used by an academic medical center in the Midwest. Of note is the absence of quantitative criteria. The center reviews quantitative criteria separately in the decision-making process. This enables its decision makers to fully assess the financial impact of alternative project portfolio decisions and the potential financial impact of collective decisions.

Criteria Weighting

Because evaluating qualitative criteria often consumes a disproportionate amount of time in the decision-making process, many organizations find it helpful to establish a scoring system that weights such criteria. An organization's capital management council should be responsible for developing such a system, and council members must explicitly agree on the criteria and weighting. Qualitative criteria are always organization specific.

Weightings may change as the organization's priorities change. For example, one organization increased the weighting labeled "fit with the strategic plan" to strengthen the importance of initiatives that mapped to its recently revised long-term plan.

In some organizations, the individuals proposing projects to the council are responsible for qualitative assessment using weighted criteria and for presenting

Outcomes and Satisfaction

How important is this project to patient clinical outcomes?
How important is this project to physician, employee, and patient experience and satisfaction?

Operating Efficiency

Will this project result in the following types of efficiencies, and can these efficiencies be quantified?

- Improved patient throughput
- Decreased length of stay and preventable readmissions
- Seamless patient care transitions
- Enhanced team-based care
- Decreased administrative burden

Infrastructure Quality

Will this project improve the appearance or functionality of existing sites of care and access to these sites?
Will the project improve the availability or timeliness of critical information (e.g., information technology)?
Will the project increase the level of coordination between the organization and its partners (e.g., physician practices, payers, employers, post-acute facilities, a medical school or its university)?

Competitive Position

Will the project have a positive impact on critical stakeholders?
Will the project result in increased market share or strengthen the organization's network of referrals?
Will the investment solidify the organization's position as a preferred provider in area networks?
Will the project improve the organization's brand and reputation?

Source: Kaufman, Hall & Associates, LLC. Used with permission.

their findings to the council. In other organizations, the council performs the qualitative assessment following review and presentation of all projects. Exhibit 6.13 shows how one hospital's capital management council defined the criteria and their relative weights. Some organizations successfully combine these two approaches, with both project sponsors and the council performing qualitative assessments.

Exhibit 6.13 Qualitative Criteria and Criteria Weighting Example

Criterion	Weighting
Safety and quality	30%
Customer value	20%
Physician alignment	20%
Process improvement	15%
Growth of mission	10%
Innovation	5%

While the criteria and weightings will differ for each organization, it is important to reiterate that financial return should not be included on this qualitative list. As stated earlier, this exclusion allows decision makers to separate the purely quantitative and objective context of the NPV analysis from the subjective and qualitative factors.

After completing the quantitative and qualitative analyses described in this chapter, an organization's capital management council is properly equipped to select a high-quality portfolio of threshold capital projects.

IMPLEMENTATION CONSIDERATIONS

First-class analysis is the backbone of effective capital allocation, especially as it relates to threshold capital initiatives. Common breakdowns in the quantitative analysis of projects include the following:

- *Incompletely quantifying the capital necessary to maintain the proposed investment after initial investment*: Examples include insufficiently recapitalizing investments in long-lived facilities and information technology upgrades.
- *Overestimating the incremental impact of an investment by exaggerating the cash flow at risk*: One example is assuming that 100 percent of the procedures associated with a replacement piece of imaging equipment are incremental, implying that if the investment was not made, 100 percent of the existing business would evaporate. This is rarely the case, although the "do nothing" scenario will result in some degradation of existing business.
- *Using a hurdle rate equal to the organization's cost of debt rather than its weighted average cost of capital*: Project-to-project evaluations will be relatively unaffected when a *consistent* hurdle rate is applied. On the other hand, the

overall value creation of the approved capital portfolio would be overstated and potentially lead to implementation of a diluted portfolio of project investments.

- *Applying an inappropriate terminal value*: One example is assuming a perpetuity growth terminal value on a piece of imaging equipment that will likely lose clinical efficacy over a five- to ten-year horizon.

Although a project's sponsor should "own" development of the financial analysis, the organization's finance team must review all prepared analyses to ensure consistency and integrity.

REFERENCES

Kaufman, K. 2006. *Best-Practice Financial Management: Six Key Concepts for Healthcare Leaders*, 3rd ed. Chicago: Health Administration Press.

National Research Council. 2005. *The Owner's Role in Project Risk Management*. Washington, DC: National Academy of Sciences.

Wilkinson, J. 2013. "Capital Budgeting Methods." The Strategic CFO. Published July 23. http://strategiccfo.com/capital-budgeting-methods-2.

CHAPTER 7

Selecting Threshold Capital Projects Using a Portfolio Approach

THIS CHAPTER DESCRIBES an approach to selecting threshold capital projects that many leading health systems have implemented successfully. The approach enables organizations to combine the information they obtain through quantitative and qualitative analyses (described in chapter 6) to select a portfolio of threshold capital projects that balances margin and mission as closely as possible. The steps in the selection process include quantitatively ranking projects, integrating qualitative data, and then uniting both analyses to make a final selection of threshold capital projects.

QUANTITATIVE PROJECT RANKING

The traditional corporate finance–based approach to project selection employs a purely quantitative view. Projects are ranked as follows: the project with the highest net present value (NPV) or expected net present value (ENPV) first, followed by projects of lesser NPV or ENPV in descending order.

Using this approach, all projects with a positive NPV or ENPV whose total capital costs do not exceed the defined capital constraint would be selected; projects that are lower on the list after the capital constraint has been exceeded, as well as projects with a negative NPV or ENPV, would not be approved. Ranking projects by NPV has been a core practice of corporate-style capital allocation and management since the 1950s.

In healthcare organizations, especially not-for-profit healthcare organizations, use of financial return as the sole decision-making criterion is rare. Most healthcare organizations add several other criteria to financial return as the basis for capital allocation decisions. The weighting of these criteria varies among organizations and often is more implicit than explicit. Some organizations establish a weighting system that effectively combines quantitative and qualitative analyses to capture mission, strategy, and financial issues in a composite ranking. This practice is recommended.

Organizations with an effective decision-making process highlight the financial implications of qualitatively driven (i.e., subjective) decisions by maintaining a list of all proposed projects in a table sorted in descending order of NPV or ENPV. By maintaining such a table, the projected financial impact of alternative allocation decisions remains transparent and allows the organization to consider the list as a portfolio of investments, as described later in this chapter. As each set of projects is approved, the council can determine whether the potential investment portfolio has a positive or a negative NPV, thereby adding to or detracting from the organization's long-term value.

The integrity of the quantitative financial analysis should be maintained throughout the decision-making process because the quantitative analysis is the benchmark against which alternative portfolios of approved capital are evaluated. Accordingly, financial return should *not* be included among the criteria used in the subjective part of the evaluation process, as mentioned in chapter 6. Including financial return dilutes the ultimate impact of this key measure of project success.

Exhibit 7.1 shows one organization's project ranking list. In this example, the total portfolio NPV of the top 11 proposed projects, sorted solely on the basis of NPV, is $34.2 million. The capital investment required to fund this portfolio is within the organization's $16 million capital constraint. This corporate finance–based allocation should represent the starting point and, more important, the benchmark against which the returns of alternative portfolios are assessed.

INTEGRATING QUALITATIVE INFORMATION

In chapter 6, an organization's capital management council identified qualitative criteria for project evaluation and assigned appropriate weightings to each criterion (see exhibit 6.13). Once the council has ranked all of the proposed projects by NPV, it can integrate these qualitative factors into its decision making.

To do so, council members vote individually on the proposed projects (15 projects in our example, itemized in exhibit 7.1). The combined voting scores establish each project's weighted qualitative ranking within the total portfolio of potential projects under consideration (exhibit 7.2). This ranking may be considerably

Exhibit 7.1 Ranking Projects by Quantitative (NPV) Score

Project	Cost	NPV ($ in thousands)	
1. Project A	$500,000	$5,400	
2. Project B	2,500,000	5,200	
3. Project C	1,000,000	5,000	
4. Project D	1,400,000	4,500	$16 million capital constraint
5. Project E	1,500,000	4,200	
6. Project F	2,250,000	3,600	
7. Project G	1,500,000	3,600	
8. Project H	600,000	1,500	
9. Project I	1,250,000	500	
10. Project J	750,000	400	
11. Project K	2,000,000	300	Portfolio NPV totals $34.2 million
12. Project L	5,000,000	0	
13. Project M	1,250,000	(750)	
14. Project N	750,000	(900)	
15. Project O	3,000,000	(2,500)	
	$25,250,000		

Source: Kaufman, Hall & Associates, LLC. Used with permission.

different from the NPV ranking illustrated in exhibit 7.1. In fact, it is possible that projects with negative NPVs will appear at the top of the list.

As shown in exhibit 7.2, the inclusion of projects with lower NPVs (including those with negative NPVs) in the capital constraint reduces the overall NPV for the portfolio of projects from $34.2 million to $27.4 million. If the council selects projects based solely on qualitative criteria, which is not the recommended approach, it would forgo about $7 million in future return (i.e., cash flow generated from projects with higher returns), which could have been used to support future strategic investment.

Organizations that do not have a structured capital decision-making process in place have actually made such decisions, preferring qualitative rankings to quantitative ones. The lack of a process also prevents the rest of the organization from seeing the impact of these decisions. With visibility into the process, the broader management team or the board may not wish to reduce the organization's ability to invest the forgone NPV of $7 million in future years.

In organizations with a best-practice process, these decisions are made consciously and communicated transparently to the entire organization. If the capital

Exhibit 7.2 Ranking Projects by Qualitative Score

Project	Cost	NPV ($ in thousands)	Qualitative Score	
1. Project D	$1,400,000	$4,500	100	
2. Project N	750,000	(900)	98	
3. Project A	500,000	5,400	92	
4. Project B	2,500,000	5,200	88	$16 million capital constraint
5. Project M	1,250,000	(750)	85	
6. Project C	1,000,000	5,000	82	
7. Project E	1,500,000	4,200	80	
8. Project F	2,250,000	3,600	78	
9. Project G	1,500,000	3,600	76	
10. Project O	3,000,000	(2,500)	71	
11. Project H	600,000	1,500	68	Portfolio NPV totals $27.4 million
12. Project J	750,000	400	63	
13. Project I	1,250,000	500	59	
14. Project K	2,000,000	300	55	
15. Project L	5,000,000	0	52	
	$25,250,000			

Source: Kaufman, Hall & Associates, LLC. Used with permission.

management council approves a capital portfolio with reduced economic benefit to the organization, it has to justify this decision.

BALANCING MARGIN AND MISSION

Best-practice capital decision making involves balancing margin and mission—the quantitative and qualitative factors assessed up to this point. This balancing might be difficult financially and politically. The key to appropriate allocation decision making lies in taking a portfolio approach with three critical, and often conflicting, objectives:

1. To protect the organization's mission and community initiatives
2. To quantify the potential impact of qualitatively based decisions
3. To ensure that total capital investment will generate sufficient returns and cash flows to both meet the organization's short-term needs and create long-term value

An organization's decision-making process must provide a structure for the portfolio review and comparison process, focusing on areas of inconsistency between qualitative and quantitative evaluation. The council must quantify the value of a proposed capital portfolio to assess the organization's ability to meet the proposed portfolio's capital requirements. The council needs a means to assess, in real time, the impact of proposed changes to the portfolio.

To focus on areas of inconsistency, the council can place, side by side, the qualitatively and quantitatively ranked lists of the projects that could be approved within the capital constraint (see exhibit 7.3). Although 15 projects originally were submitted, only 11 now appear in the quantitative ranking and 10 appear in the qualitative ranking. The council eliminated from further consideration Project L, which had the lowest NPV and a low qualitative score. Seven projects (A through G) appear on both lists because they met both quantitative and qualitative criteria. These projects should not require further discussion; the council should allocate capital to these seven. In fact, council discussion should focus on the seven projects—H, I, J, K, M, N, and O—that appear on only one of the lists.

As exhibit 7.4 illustrates, nearly $10.7 million of the total $16 million threshold capital constraint will be allocated to projects A through G, which have a portfolio NPV of $27 million. This means that only about $5.4 million in threshold capital

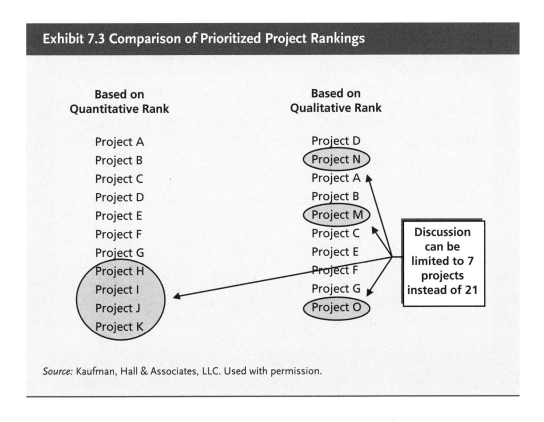

Exhibit 7.3 Comparison of Prioritized Project Rankings

Source: Kaufman, Hall & Associates, LLC. Used with permission.

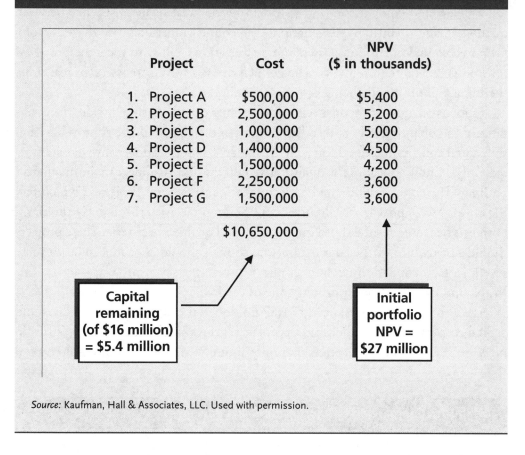

Exhibit 7.4 Projects Meeting Both Quantitative and Qualitative Criteria

Project	Cost	NPV ($ in thousands)
1. Project A	$500,000	$5,400
2. Project B	2,500,000	5,200
3. Project C	1,000,000	5,000
4. Project D	1,400,000	4,500
5. Project E	1,500,000	4,200
6. Project F	2,250,000	3,600
7. Project G	1,500,000	3,600
	$10,650,000	

Capital remaining (of $16 million) = $5.4 million

Initial portfolio NPV = $27 million

Source: Kaufman, Hall & Associates, LLC. Used with permission.

remains for the other seven projects under consideration. Furthermore, because the NPV for projects A through G is $27 million, the remaining projects under discussion could have a combined negative NPV—of up to $27 million—and still create a balanced portfolio.

In this example, no combination of remaining projects could create such a negative NPV. The lowest NPV possible, given the remaining available capital constraint and the projects under discussion, is negative $4.2 million. Regardless, the council should approve additional projects that minimize the negative economic consequences for the organization.

How should the council allocate the remaining $5.4 million? Exhibit 7.5 shows that the total investment required for all seven remaining projects—$9.6 million— exceeds the available capital, so the council clearly needs to make some choices. Selecting the projects with the highest qualitative scores—M, N, and O—would not exceed the available capital but would result in reducing the portfolio's total NPV by more than $4 million. Selecting the projects with positive NPVs—H, I, J,

Exhibit 7.5 Remaining Projects for Threshold Capital Allocation

Project	Cost	NPV ($ in thousands)	Qualitative Score
1. Project H	$600,000	$1,500	68
2. Project I	1,250,000	500	59
3. Project J	750,000	400	63
4. Project K	2,000,000	300	55
5. Project M	1,250,000	(750)	85
6. Project N	750,000	(900)	98
7. Project O	3,000,000	(2,500)	71
	$9,600,000		

Source: Kaufman, Hall & Associates, LLC. Used with permission.

and K—also would not exceed available capital and would contribute $2.7 million to the portfolio's NPV.

Either decision could be supported, given the strength of the seven projects in the portfolio that met both the quantitative and qualitative criteria. Nonetheless, the final selection should be made in a transparent way that enables management to reinforce its support for all aspects of the organization's strategy.

As described in chapter 2, the organization's capital management council is the linchpin to an effective process for allocating and managing capital, especially as it relates to threshold capital projects. Strong, centralized management seeks to discourage conditions under which the allocation of capital devolves into a free-for-all. Political clout, timing (first to the trough), and access to senior management must not influence decision making; decisions must be based on a true analysis of what optimizes the strategic and financial strength of the organization.

Chapter 8 describes the process used by the council to continuously manage the capital process after it selects a portfolio of threshold capital projects.

IMPLEMENTATION CONSIDERATIONS

A portfolio view is both the means and the end to a best-practice capital management process. Batch evaluation of potential threshold capital projects supports a holistic view of potential investments and ultimately positions an organization to most appropriately balance margin and mission.

The meeting at which the capital management council approves threshold capital projects is often viewed as the apex of the capital decision-making process. Executives on the council must be in a position to make effective decisions across the portfolio of potential threshold capital projects. Considerations include the following:

- Collect, organize, and distribute the breadth of quantitative and qualitative information in a manner and format that are both consistent and comparable across the variety of potential projects and easily consumed by the capital management council.
- Allow sufficient time (at least one week) for the council to review the materials before the meeting.
- Consider gathering each council member's input regarding the qualitative ranking of the portfolio in advance of the meeting.
- Structure the meeting to move at an efficient pace by requiring that council members fully review the premeeting materials and ensuring that no critical information is withheld. Less than five minutes per project for follow-up questions and clarification should be sufficient.
- Set the expectation that the meeting and process for approving threshold capital projects will be completed in one sitting and in no more than a full day.

Managing the Postallocation Process

A BEST-PRACTICE CAPITAL management process does not end when allocation decisions are made. Rather, the postallocation process commences. This process includes reviewing and revalidating projects before their actual funding, making decisions regarding the timing of capital spending, handling any budget deficits or surpluses that occur, monitoring capital spending on an ongoing basis, and determining the appropriate course of action based on performance results. A discussion of these topics follows.

FUNDING REVIEW AND REVALIDATION

Best-practice capital management requires some form of revalidation of project parameters before final funding of allocated capital. Revalidation ensures that new data or information obtained following the project's approval can be considered and integrated appropriately.

Many organizations require project sponsors to update their original request for threshold capital to support the revalidation process. For these organizations, using a standardized format for capital requests helps to ensure that sponsors provide the information needed for decision making at the time of both allocation and revalidation. The same data and analysis that supported the original allocation decision will support the project's revalidation at the time of funding. Some of the project's parameters may have changed in the period since the capital request was initially evaluated. Information captured through the standardized format enables such changes to be identified and evaluated.

Some organizations consider allocation decisions to be unalterable. In these organizations, all approved projects receive funding. Other organizations are willing to revisit allocation decisions when project sponsors seek funding for approved projects. In suboptimal cases, an organization makes allocation decisions and funding decisions separately, resulting in two different allocation and approval processes. In this situation, a project sponsor shepherds the project through the structured batch allocation process before the start of the year but has no assurance that allocated capital ultimately will be made available. This scenario undermines the integrity of the initial allocation decision, extends decision-making time frames, and increases the potential for politics to creep back into the decision process. Clearly, these results are not desirable.

The revalidation process must reaffirm, based on updated information, that the project for which capital has been allocated remains essentially the same. In a best-practice allocation process, threshold capital requests (projects with costs above a defined dollar level) undergo an analytically rigorous review at the time of allocation decision making. Similarly, rigorous revalidation before funding also typically occurs with threshold capital requests. The capital management council is responsible for this revalidation function.

Exhibit 8.1 illustrates how revalidation fits into an integrated process. At some point following the initial allocation of capital, the project sponsor initiates the revalidation process by submitting a request to obtain actual project funding. This funding request is submitted during the fiscal year for which the allocation has been made (the allocation year), but the specific timing will vary by project and by organization. In some cases, the council revalidates the project at the point of contract execution, but in other cases the council revalidates it earlier, such as when detailed drawings for a new construction project are finalized. To some extent, timing is a function of organizational culture. Some organizational councils require complete information to approve funding; other councils allow sponsors to finalize projects within broad, but defined, parameters. With either approach, the council assumes responsibility for moving the funding request forward.

Decision Making Related to Postapproval Project Costs

The scope of revalidation for approved threshold capital projects must be well defined. Through the allocation decision-making process, the capital management council has already confirmed the project's strategic necessity and economic appropriateness. The revalidation process should not be viewed as another chance

Exhibit 8.1 Decision Flow from Postallocation to Funding Approval

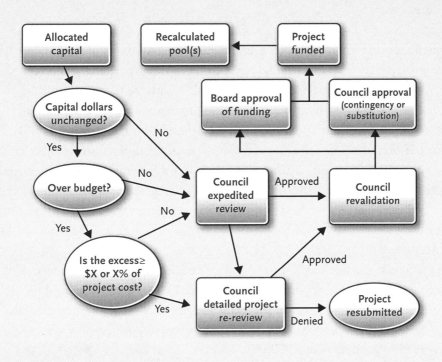

Source: Kaufman, Hall & Associates, LLC. Used with permission.

to take a shot at the project's legitimacy. Rather, revalidation should verify that the project's original premise remains sound; that the key assumptions continue to be supported; and, most important, that the project's investment requirements remain consistent with the original request.

If the project's investment requirements have *not changed*, or if they have decreased, the project remains valid. If the costs have *decreased*, the council should validate the new cost figure and return the unneeded funds to the organizational contingency pool for future application as determined by the council. If the repatriated dollars are significant, the council can also decide to allocate some of those dollars to the project that was designated as the next priority on the list of potential projects (compiled through the process described in chapter 7) but for which no allocation was originally made. Alternatively, the council could decide to retain the dollars as balance sheet reserves, potentially increasing the organization's capital constraint in the subsequent year.

If project costs have *increased*, and the increase is material (as defined for that organization's process), the council should review the project carefully. Three scenarios are possible:

1. The higher investment needed undermines the economics of the project. The project's costs may have increased to the point where the projected return on investment (ROI) has been eliminated or reduced below that of the next most worthy project. In some organizations, the council halts project funding pending the project's reconfiguration to improve its ROI. In other organizations, the council simply declines to fund the project at the time of revalidation. Again, this decision is a function of organizational culture. Projects whose funding is declined through the revalidation process can be resubmitted for allocation the following year, assuming the questions regarding the reliability and validity of the project's cost assumptions are fully addressed.

2. Project costs have increased, but they are within an approved, preestablished range. For example, one community hospital with a capital threshold defined at $500,000 also identifies the allowable range for project cost increases as 10 percent of original project costs. If a threshold capital project that was originally projected to have costs of $800,000 has revalidated costs of $840,000, the council moves the project forward for funding approval and allocates dollars from the contingency pool to cover the additional $40,000 in project costs. Should contingency dollars not be available, the council would have to decide whether to stop the project or to fund it by deferring another project.

3. Project costs have increased beyond the preestablished range, but they are not high enough to negatively affect the project's ROI. Because the council previously approved the project's strategic necessity and appropriateness, it moves the project forward for funding and works to determine the source of the required additional capital.

As with the original allocation process, the revalidation process in no way diminishes the board's role in approving projects for capital funding. If anything, this best-practice structure improves the board's ability to perform its duties. When the capital management council brings a specific, revalidated capital project to the board for funding approval, the board has the assurance that the council has thoroughly and consistently analyzed the project, has identified it as a priority strategic investment for the organization, and has vetted it for any material changes that would affect the direction of the original allocation (budgeting) decision. The board, of course, will already have seen the project as part of the recommended capital budget and will be aware of its imminent need for funding. The board will also have a complete understanding of the project's funding source, including whether the project is using funds from the contingency pool.

TIMING OF CAPITAL SPENDING

The capital management council also manages the overall schedule for funding allocated threshold capital projects. The organization's finance team should support this function by providing the council with anticipated cash flow schedules on a quarterly basis, accompanied by a year-to-date statement of operating cash flows and their variance from the financial plan or budget.

In some organizations, the council also manages *nonthreshold* capital spending by releasing nonthreshold dollars on a quarterly basis subject to the organization's achievement of agreed-upon operating performance levels. This degree of oversight is less common, especially in multihospital systems, but it does permit corporate-level management of spending to ensure that operating performance appropriately matches capital expenditure levels. It also helps to ensure that the organization does not run out of available nonthreshold capital dollars before year-end.

One approach to the management of the nonthreshold pool is to release only a portion of the total dollars allocated in each of the first three quarters. Assuming the council meets on a quarterly basis, this method is manageable and allows the council to increase the size of the nonthreshold capital pool in the event the organization's performance is significantly better than anticipated in the financial plan that formed the basis for the capital constraint.

Management of *threshold* capital projects is more straightforward. At the time of allocation, the council will have ranked the threshold capital projects—according to both quantitative and qualitative factors—and will have built a related cash flow schedule covering the upcoming allocation year. Thus, the council can proactively manage the release of funds for spending (subject to any board funding approval requirements) based on the original project ranking and anticipated project timing.

The cash flow schedule for project investments should reflect the organization's current and projected cash flow position by fiscal quarter. In addition, the cash flow projections must be continually updated to control the release of cash for capital projects as a function of organizational performance. In this way, the council can use actual quarterly operating cash flow results to drive the release of funds as follows:

- If operating cash flow is *below* plan, the implementation of approved threshold and nonthreshold capital projects should be proportionately reduced. Threshold capital reductions would begin with the lowest-ranked projects scheduled for the last quarter.
- If operating cash flow *exceeds* plan, options available to the council include
  - approving additional threshold capital in the fourth quarter;
  - approving increased nonthreshold capital levels for subsequent quarters; or
  - retaining the cash on the organization's balance sheet to carry over to the next year and, all other things being equal, resulting in an increased capital constraint in the coming year.

If the council determines that the organization has insufficient capital capacity because operating performance is significantly below the target established in both the financial planning and operating budget processes, the spending on threshold capital projects may need to be deferred to a later quarter or even into the subsequent year. Any such changes to initial allocations or project timing should be based on review of the organization's or operating unit's financial performance relative to the financial plan on which the capital constraint was based.

Midyear financial performance is particularly critical because, at the end of two full quarters, a true picture of the organization's current-year financial trajectory can be developed. At midyear, the council can best determine whether the organization's funding needs and capital availability are in balance. If they are not in balance, the council should be empowered to make appropriate adjustments to third-quarter and fourth-quarter spending.

Handling Deferred Capital Spending

The council also should establish a policy for handling capital that has been allocated but has been deferred because of adjustments made to improve organizational operating performance. An example of such a policy follows:

- When the council defers nonthreshold capital spending because the organization has insufficient capital capacity, the operating unit's management team has the authority to fund the spending through the subsequent year's nonthreshold capital allocation pool or through the threshold capital review process, as appropriate.
- Threshold capital projects that are deferred by the council because it has determined the organization has insufficient capital capacity will be

considered carryforward capital and will be managed under the policy governing that type of capital as part of the subsequent year's capital management process.

Deferral of capital spending because of underperformance is a serious issue with serious consequences. As reflected in these policy statements, best-practice capital management does not give a deferred threshold capital request an analytical pass; no tacit approval or additional capital is made available to fund these capital items. They essentially become part of the standard capital management process in the subsequent year. The underlying reason for the deferral—underperformance—must be acknowledged and addressed.

UNSPENT ALLOCATED CAPITAL

On occasion, threshold capital projects may not require as much funding as was projected at the time of allocation. This situation may become evident when funding approval is sought (i.e., when the project is revalidated) or when the project is completed. The capital management council's policies should address unspent capital for both threshold and nonthreshold capital projects. Such policies will ensure that departments within a hospital, or hospitals within a system, do not revert to the political allocation of leftover funds and convert funds allocated for one purpose to another purpose beyond the purview of the capital process.

Policies related to unspent allocated capital should address the following:

- At the conclusion of a threshold capital project, unspent capital should not be transferred to another project or spent in any other manner. This allocated capital must be returned to the contingency pool to be reallocated in either the current year or future years, as determined by the council.
- Allocated nonthreshold capital that has not been spent at the conclusion of a fiscal year should not be carried forward to the subsequent year. Rather, the allocated dollars should be returned to the organizational balance sheet, mitigating the need to build cash-reserve levels and increasing the subsequent year's capital constraint.

For example, a department manager who receives approval in October for a $500,000 project determines in July of the following year that the contracts required for the initiative total only $450,000. The manager returns $50,000 to the capital pool for reallocation as either threshold or nonthreshold capital, as determined by the council.

Some organizations may be concerned that the nonthreshold policy discussed here creates a "use it or lose it" mentality because the policy essentially says that unspent nonthreshold capital allocated to an operating unit will revert to the organization at year-end. These concerns can be alleviated by permitting controlled carryforward of nonthreshold capital for spending in the first quarter of the following year. Of course, it is always in the organization's best interest to minimize the amount of nonthreshold capital carried forward. The more significant this carryforward becomes, the more difficult it is to establish a finite capital constraint. The nonthreshold carryforward essentially becomes a contingent liability; there is no way to know what portion of it will ultimately be spent.

EMERGENCY AND OFF-CYCLE CAPITAL REQUESTS

A best-practice capital management process provides for emergency capital and off-cycle capital requests that can be considered outside of the annual batch process and specifies the required approval procedures for such capital items. However, the process design should define these types of requests in a way that limits their number and frequency. In addition, such requests should never be exempted from the rigor and discipline required during the annual batch process. For example, a children's hospital outlined the following policy:

- *Emergency capital* is defined as unanticipated capital needs for facility code violations or equipment failures that materially affect a core business or the quality of patient care. The associated policy is as follows:
  - Nonthreshold emergency capital follows the decentralized capital authorization process, with funding through substitution(s) or from contingency reserves at the department or operating unit level.
  - Threshold emergency capital requires council approval, with funding from the organization's contingency pool or through threshold capital project substitution, as necessary and as determined by the council.
- *Off-cycle capital* is defined as nonemergent and truly unforeseen capital needs that management believes cannot wait for the next planning cycle. The policy includes the same review, approval, and funding processes as with emergency capital.

In a successful capital allocation and management process, emergency and off-cycle capital needs should be relatively rare, and the capital management council's policy should not encourage such requests. The council should promptly and consistently deny any requests for off-cycle capital from individuals who are trying to "game" the process by claiming off-cycle status for capital needs that were (or should have been) known and exceed the available allocation. In addition, no off-cycle, incremental threshold or nonthreshold capital should be allocated to operating units that spend their allocated capital before year-end, unless the council has complete confidence that a specific request for emergency or off-cycle capital is valid.

APPLICATION OF CONTINGENCY DOLLARS

The capital management council should have sole authority over the use of contingency capital, the amount of which is defined each year as part of the calculation of net cash flow available for capital spending (the capital constraint, described in chapter 3). Use of the contingency capital pool should be reserved for emergency and off-cycle capital requests, funding of budget overruns, and support of the organization's vital capital needs if the organization's financial performance falls short of planned levels.

The council should define a specific time each fiscal year—typically the end of the second quarter—to assess financial performance (i.e., profitability and cash flow) and the possible need to release contingency pool dollars to either the threshold or the nonthreshold pool. For example, if the organization's financial performance is at or above plan at the end of the second quarter, the council (and only the council) should have the discretion to release contingency dollars. Such release would clearly be based on comprehensive cash flow projections and review of outstanding, potential threshold capital needs.

CONTINUOUS PROJECT MONITORING

Postapproval review and monitoring are vital to the integrity of the capital management process. Successful organizations require definition of quantifiable indicators of a project's success as part of the project's business plan, measure performance against these indicators, and devise and implement plans to remedy lower-than-anticipated performance.

Ongoing measurement of actual investment performance must be built into both the governance and the calendar of the capital management process. Such measurement provides credibility, enabling the comparison of actual results with projected results. Postallocation monitoring helps ensure that cost and revenue projections are both on target and reasonable. Furthermore, with measurement against preestablished parameters, individuals can be held accountable for performance results. The presence of ongoing monitoring ultimately improves the quality of up-front analysis and helps ensure realistic projections and assumptions. Knowing that a project's performance will be reviewed and the project's champion will be held accountable keeps managers and executives from providing overly aggressive or unsupported cash flow estimates in submitted business plans.

Ongoing measurement also allows the rest of the organization to learn about an investment's success or failure. It creates an historical track record and corporate memory, and it also provides lessons learned about different types of projects and how they performed relative to expectations. This record enables executives to better evaluate assumptions the next time a similar project is brought to the council for consideration.

The capital management council should define the time frame for postallocation and continued funding review of every approved threshold capital project. For example, one organization established the following guidelines:

> The council will review each threshold capital project annually until the project has been operational for one full year following completion. Council review includes completed projects that are operational in the first investment year as well as multiyear projects that are not operational in the first investment year.

In this organization, projects with a long build-out or start-up period could be required to undergo annual reviews for several years.

Postallocation, retrospective analysis should mirror the prospective analysis prepared in support of the original capital request. Postallocation benchmarks and metrics, both qualitative and quantitative, should be based on the benchmarks and metrics used in the project's business plan.

In fact, it is appropriate to employ a standardized project tracking form that is structured identically to the capital request form used by the council to make allocation decisions. The point of such standardization is that benchmarks become more distinct, quantifiable, and measurable when a project's sponsor understands that any assumption made in support of the business plan projections will be a metric used for performance evaluation. From an organizational standpoint, this means better up-front analysis and better capability to manage and assess postallocation performance.

RESPONDING TO PERFORMANCE RESULTS

Best-practice capital monitoring requires more than simply developing data collection and analysis requirements. Organizations also must determine what they are going to do with information about a project that is not meeting performance targets established in the business plan. Can the project be improved? Should it be delayed or halted? Assumptions about related or similar projects may also need to be revised.

Organizational leaders must foster an understanding that not all projects for which capital is allocated will be successful. Because this is an axiom of business planning, every project request must include specific metrics that define the point at which the "plug is pulled" on an underperforming investment, as well as the specific exit strategy that will be implemented.

The consistency, frequency, and sophistication of postallocation project review and validation of projected returns from capital investments vary considerably among organizations. Many healthcare organizations wait far too long to either modify or terminate a bad capital investment decision.

A survey of some of the nation's most sophisticated health systems indicated that many systems are only just beginning to develop and implement processes to monitor returns against expected investment performance, even though they have operated a structured capital management process for some time (Sussman 2016). Some systems perform feasibility updates or retrospective reviews approximately one year after a project has been completed and is operational, regardless of when it was approved. Chief financial officers at the hospital units typically perform the postallocation analyses, which are then reviewed at the system level by corporate finance staff. In some healthcare organizations, the review process's lack of consistency, standardization, and comprehensiveness diminishes its ability to enhance and inform decision making.

To give the postapproval process "teeth," the capital management council should consider the following strategies:

- Require review of all approved projects for at least three years following allocation, which for projects with an extended period until start-up would include at least the first full year of the projects' operations.
- Require retrospective review of randomly selected projects at different stages of their completion.
- Require retrospective review of all approved projects as a prerequisite to submitting capital requests in the subsequent year's capital management process.

- Share the retrospective review directly with the organization's board.
- Create a direct link between capital approval and the operating budget. (Allocation of capital predicated on achieving operating efficiencies should result in direct and specific reductions in departmental operating budgets.)

An organization's disciplined use of a best-practice postallocation process supports the rigor of its overall capital management process. Having a multiyear strategy for implementing a best-practice process, including ongoing education and communication about the process (discussed in chapter 9), ensures that the capital management process is thoroughly integrated with the organization's ongoing planning and decision-making processes.

COMPREHENSIVE CAPITAL BUDGET MANAGEMENT

In addition to the project-specific postallocation monitoring that has been the focus of this chapter, monitoring and management of the entire allocated capital budget is a vital organizational process.

In a best-practice process, management of *nonthreshold* capital spending against funds released by the capital management council is decentralized and falls under the purview of the departmental, entity, or regional managers to whom the original allocation of nonthreshold funds was made.

The capital management council has the responsibility to monitor and manage the overall status of the annual dollars allocated from the *threshold* capital pool. To some extent, this function represents classic budget-variance reporting. However, given the project-based nature of threshold capital, some additional data are required to enable the capital management council to proactively manage the organization's capital outlays from the threshold capital pool.

Exhibit 8.2 illustrates the type of report for threshold capital projects that should be generated from the organization's capital planning and management software. This report should derive from the same database that supported the capital allocation process to ensure that project parameters and approvals are consistent across the entire process. Reported on a frequent, periodic basis (e.g., monthly), the information included in this report is intended to provide the capital management council with a comprehensive view of threshold capital pool status including the following:

1. *Original budget*: Identifies project dollars that were allocated (and board approved) during the annual one-batch decision-making process
2. *Transfers*: Reflects amounts approved to be added to or subtracted from the original project allocation by the authority of the capital management council through (1) the revalidation process; (2) use or return of dollars to the contingency pool; or (3) substitution of an emergency or out-of-cycle threshold project for a different project originally included in the allocation.
3. *Purchase requests*: Amounts that have been approved for funding for which purchase orders have been issued, but that have not yet been invoiced by the vendors.
4. *Actual*: Reflects the amount that has been spent on a project-to-date basis.
5. *Committed*: Total project encumbrances, including actual expenditures, purchase requests outstanding, and amounts that have been approved for funding and that are in the organization's purchasing process for issuance of a purchase order.

For accurate threshold project management and monitoring, inclusion in this report of information related to funds not yet spent, but committed (i.e., the data on purchase requests and committed) is vital and reflects a departure from standard variance reporting. This additional information gives the capital management council a clearer line of sight into the comprehensive status of the project and expands their ability to be proactive in managing project spending.

For example, in exhibit 8.2, the last threshold project, Master Facility Plan, New Cancer Center, has a budget of about $11.1 million. Actual expenditures of approximately $2 million have been incurred to date. In a standard variance management process, this would be the full extent of reporting, creating a management view that $9.1 million remains available to be spent on the project. However, for threshold projects that are large and can span extended periods of time, such as the New Cancer Center, standard reporting falls short. In the case of the New Cancer Center, purchase requests of $360,000 and other commitments of $110,000 working their way through the purchasing process have already encumbered project funds. As a result, only $8.6 million of the originally allocated project funding is available.

With knowledge of the additional $470,000 of encumbrance, the capital management council has a clearer picture of the project's status. In addition, as the fiscal year comes to an end, this type of reporting will provide a more accurate quantification of carryforward capital needs and their impact on the calculation of the subsequent years' capital constraint (see chapter 3).

Exhibit 8.2 Comprehensive Capital Management Report

Department	Project Description/ Transaction Notes	Original Budget	Budget Exceptions	Transfers	Adjusted Budget	Purchase Requests	Committed	Remaining Funds	Actual
19000	Land Purchase, for New MOB	0	1,000,000	1,000,000	1,000,000	0	0	1,000,000	0
	Transfer TO project (2016.001.19000.001) FROM project (Contingency)			1,000,000		0	0	1,000,000	0
19000	Contingency, Main Campus Contingency Pool	4,105,000	0	(1,134,250)	2,970,750	0	0	2,970,750	0
	Transfer FROM project (Contingency) TO project (2016.001.19000.001)			(1,000,000)		0	0		0
	Transfer FROM project (Contingency) TO project (2016.001.27370.001)			(60,750)		0	0		0
	Transfer FROM project (Contingency) TO project (2016.002.29530.001)			(58,000)		0	0		0
	Transfer FROM project (Contingency) TO project (2016.001.28510.001)			(15,500)		0	0		0
26750	Mammography Unit, Digital Mammo Unit	540,000	0	0	540,000	0	0	540,000	0
27370	Lift, Replacement of Existing	0	60,750	60,750	60,750	0	0	60,750	0
	Transfer TO project (2016.001.27370.001) FROM project (Contingency)			60,750		0	0		0
27400	General Construction, New Cardiac Center	14,250,000	0	0	14,250,000	0	0	14,250,000	0
27540	General Construction, Sleep Lab Expansion	1,125,000	0	0	1,125,000	0	0	1,125,000	0

27550	EMG (Spine Neuro), Cyber Knife	5,855,000	0	5,855,000	0	0	5,855,000	0
27640	General Renovation, OR Remodel	1,000,000	0	1,000,000	0	0	1,000,000	0
28510	Refrigerator, Replacement Due to Breakdown	0	15,500	15,500		0	15,500	0
	Transfer TO project (2016.001.28510.001) FROM project (Contingency)		15,500	15,500		0		0
29530	Sanitizer Unit, Replacement Due to Breakdown	0	58,000	58,000		0	58,000	0
	Transfer TO project (2016.002.29530.001) FROM project (Contingency)	58,000	58,000	58,000		0		0
102002	General Construction, Dental Surgery Expansion	968,000	0	968,000	0	0	968,000	0
26140	Bed, Bariatric Beds	48,050	0	48,050	15,550	32,500	15,550	0
	Purchase of 2 of the 3 beds currently budgeted		0		0	32,500		0
	Last of 3 beds to order		0		15,550	0		0
26480	Master Facility Plan, New Cancer Center	11,125,000	0	11,125,000	360,550	2,512,569	8,612,431	2,041,780
	Totals	39,016,050	1,134,250	39,016,050	376,100	2,512,569	36,470,981	2,041,780

Source: Kaufman, Hall & Associates, LLC. Used with permission.

IMPLEMENTATION CONSIDERATIONS

Effective processes and good decision making do not end with the capital approval decision. In fact, some of the most detailed design and implementation efforts relate to the process components that come into play *after* the capital allocation decision has been made. For this reason, organizations must carefully consider postallocation procedures to achieve a successful capital allocation and management process. Thoughtful design and implementation of postallocation procedures

- increase the accuracy and visibility of threshold capital approval decisions at the time of actual funding (as opposed to allocation) based on real-time information;
- maintain the rigor of the portfolio approach by closing (or at least limiting) all potential loopholes for project owners to circumvent the batch process;
- ensure that the highest level of rigor is applied to all threshold capital project decisions, even in limited off-cycle situations; and
- encourage the organization and accountable project owners to do what they said they would do in terms of both capital capacity and project performance.

REFERENCE

Sussman, J. H. 2016. *Survey of Capital Allocation Approaches in 26 U.S. Health Systems*. Skokie, IL: Kaufman, Hall & Associates, LLC.

CHAPTER 9

Making It Happen and Keeping It Going

THE SUCCESSFUL ROLLOUT of a high-quality capital allocation and management process requires organization-wide commitment to the process. The commitment must originate with leaders at the highest level and pervade all levels of management. Education, best-practice tools, transparent communication, and execution of a solid implementation plan with a realistic time frame, as described in this chapter, help to secure such commitment.

THE ROLE OF EDUCATION

An organization's key constituents must thoroughly understand basic corporate finance principles as well as the mechanics of the capital allocation and management process and its time frame. The entire management team should have at least a working understanding of the corporate finance concepts embodied in effective decision making. Many organizations view the capital allocation and management process strictly as a finance function, but nonfinancial managers' participation is critical for an effective process.

Much can be learned from corporate finance leaders such as General Electric, which pioneered the organization-wide application of a rigorous capital allocation and management process. At General Electric, *everybody*—from administrative assistants to senior vice presidents—knows the requirements and timing of the planning and allocation processes, including when capital project proposals must be submitted and when decisions will be made. They also know how capital requests are evaluated (i.e., the criteria that are used), which requests have been approved, and which have not. Extensive ongoing education and communication are required to achieve this exceptional level of transparency.

Education that successfully supports the capital allocation and management process has two key characteristics:

1. *The education is ongoing.* Learning about relatively new methods and concepts, especially when they will be applied only on an episodic basis, is like trying to learn a foreign language in one class. Staff members deserve, and often demand, ongoing educational opportunities to enhance their ability to analyze and present strategic capital opportunities in a manner that improves the chances that those opportunities will be approved. In some organizations, this type of education includes quarterly, semiannual, or annual sessions that review basic concepts and delve into more advanced techniques.

2. *The education uses a curriculum that teaches employees how to evaluate the strategic and financial impact of potential projects.* The curriculum must cover the methods for analyzing different types of projects. For example, how should the cost of *not* replacing assets be factored into the evaluation of an investment proposal? Is there a best-practice approach to assessing the potential cannibalization effects of a proposed project? Finally, what is the appropriate use of sensitivity analysis in assessing a proposed investment?

Many organizations fail to consistently provide the financial resources, human resources, and tools needed for appropriate and effective education. However, considering the importance and long-term impact of capital allocation and management decisions, organizations must invest in such educational resource costs. An organization clearly benefits when employees throughout the organization understand how to define a good project investment, how to prepare and present the related analysis, and how to establish and manage a project against defined measures of success.

When designing an ongoing education program, executives should consider the following questions:

- How does the organization provide staff with the education necessary to evaluate complex projects?
- How does the organization ensure that staff members have access to the right tools to perform the required analysis?
- How often should education be provided?

- How can the organization ensure that project definitions and quantitative techniques are consistently applied?
- What benchmarks can the organization use to screen out unworthy projects?

During the early years of best-practice process implementation, project sponsors' capabilities and the quality of their analytical assumptions and presentations may be inconsistent. This can create disparities in project sponsors' ability to acquire capital. A continuing, broad education effort can minimize such variation.

Some employees, particularly department-level managers, may be unfamiliar with the quantitative analytical tools used in corporate finance. These individuals may require in-depth education and training on such tools, both initially and on an ongoing basis.

The most effective way to institutionalize the best-practice capital allocation and management process is to ensure that line managers are familiar with the necessary tools and techniques to analyze capital requests. Finance staff cannot and should not be expected to perform all of the analytical work associated with capital request submissions.

Requests for capital are often generated from the "core" of a healthcare organization and frequently include clinical initiatives to improve patient care quality or increase service volume. Including clinical staff members in capital management education will empower both the clinicians and the nonclinician administrative staff members to generate valid ideas, perform the related quantitative and qualitative analyses, and effectively present their projects. This approach has two benefits; it (1) minimizes potential end runs around the process and (2) enhances overall financial knowledge.

Exhibit 9.1 presents a high-level outline of an introductory session on the capital allocation and management process for physician leaders. The session focuses on how the capital allocation and management process supports an organization's transformation to a population health, value-based model.

Because a sound capital allocation and management process relies on quantitative techniques such as net-present-value (NPV) analysis, the process must be implemented by people who have a working knowledge of the proper use of NPV, including its theory and application. Technical training must be available to anyone in the organization who may submit proposed capital projects for review. The training must be geared to educate a wide range of employees with a range of educational and occupational backgrounds, from formally trained financial analysts to self-taught departmental managers. The goal is to provide all staff members with a common language and approach to project analysis, and to ensure their continued, active participation in the process.

THE ROLE OF BEST-PRACTICE TOOLS

A software tool that can enhance the efficiency and effectiveness of the capital allocation and management process is a must-have technology asset. The tool should be designed to (1) automate and support all phases of the process for initiating, evaluating, and approving capital, and (2) monitor capital spending. This type of tool ensures that the organization has the financial context on which to base key project investment decisions, as well as evidence that the approved initiatives ultimately have met the organization's strategic and financial objectives.

A best-practice tool also should be designed to

- ensure that capital requests are submitted with consistent supporting detail and analysis, enabling comparison of projects across quantitative and qualitative measures;
- consolidate all capital requests in a central repository that becomes a single source of information from which portfolio-based decisions can be made; and
- monitor project progress and actual performance versus plan.

Exhibit 9.2 shows the types of information that should be included in a central repository and the questions leaders should ask to obtain that information.

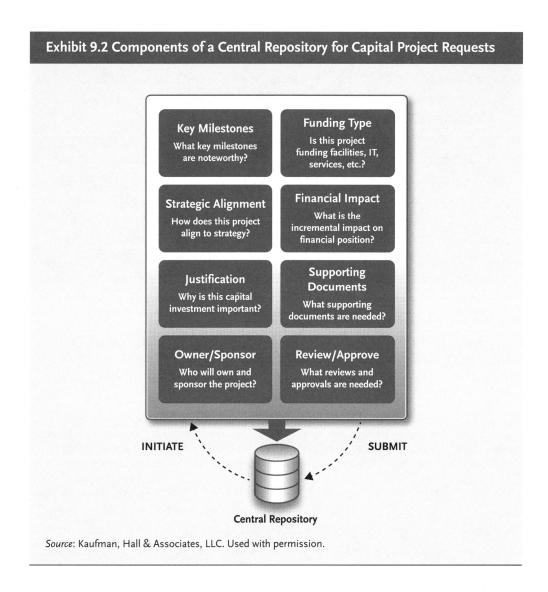

Source: Kaufman, Hall & Associates, LLC. Used with permission.

Management should ask the following big-picture questions to assess its best-practice capital allocation and management tool:

- Do we have the right templates to support a full range of requirements, from simple analysis to comprehensive business planning (e.g., market imperatives, all types of costs, incremental revenues, clinical imperatives)?
- Do the templates capture information requirements for the different stakeholders (e.g., system and local leadership, the capital council, the board of trustees)?
- What information is needed for different types of projects (e.g., major construction, clinical equipment, infrastructure, physician practices, other business acquisitions or joint ventures)?

- What level of analysis is appropriate for different types of threshold and nonthreshold initiatives (e.g., replacement of existing assets, expansion of existing programs, new services or facilities, recruitment and retention of professional staff)?

This last item in the list is critical. Leaders must recognize that although all initiatives require some level of analysis, including an estimate of the amount of capital required, certain types of initiatives—especially those that are not predicated on achieving market-based objectives (e.g., increased market share or incremental volumes)—do not require extensive market or financial research. For example, replacing existing equipment or hiring a new department chair does not require extensive market analysis to define market share, market demographics, and the like. The analysis should, however, include a specific description of the proposed investment's strategic value to the organization.

All types of investment proposals should be supported, at a minimum, by basic analysis that includes a proposed time frame for needed funding. Exhibit 9.3 illustrates the general analytic requirements associated with each type of initiative.

Support of Optimal Allocation Decisions

Organization-wide use of an online request form can guide and structure capital requests and eliminate problems associated with stand-alone spreadsheet models. For all requests gathered through the submission process, a standardized return on investment evaluation should incorporate the strategic, financial, mission-related, and operational aspects of alternative potential investments.

Organizations should use workflow tools to ensure expediency and the proper level of scrutiny and perspective throughout the review process. Automatic alerts and notifications to relevant stakeholders can facilitate prompt review and approval of capital requests.

After the proper stakeholders have reviewed a capital request and deemed it complete, it can be moved forward through the decision-making process with the confidence of knowing that all potential requirements and effects have been assessed.

The right software tool will enable rational comparisons of potential projects and initiatives through an embedded ranking and scoring system, thus supporting process consistency and transparency. Using this type of tool, the capital management council can effectively review, compare, and rank capital requests based on strategic fit, need, and priority. As a result, an organization's capital management

Exhibit 9.3 Business Analysis by Project Type

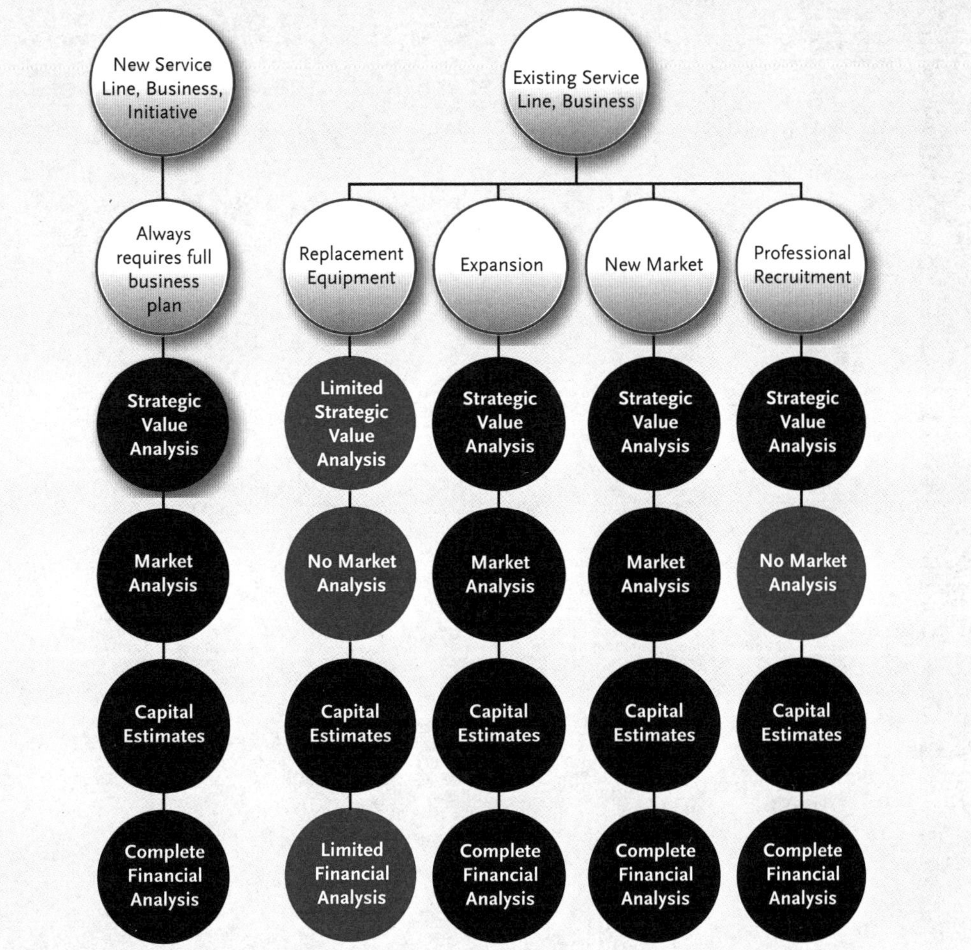

New Service Line, Business, Initiative

Existing Service Line, Business

Always requires full business plan | Replacement Equipment | Expansion | New Market | Professional Recruitment

Strategic Value Analysis | Limited Strategic Value Analysis | Strategic Value Analysis | Strategic Value Analysis | Strategic Value Analysis

Market Analysis | No Market Analysis | Market Analysis | Market Analysis | No Market Analysis

Capital Estimates | Capital Estimates | Capital Estimates | Capital Estimates | Capital Estimates

Complete Financial Analysis | Limited Financial Analysis | Complete Financial Analysis | Complete Financial Analysis | Complete Financial Analysis

Source: Kaufman, Hall & Associates, LLC. Used with permission.

council can achieve its goal of balancing the portfolio of approved projects across all areas requiring investment.

Exhibit 9.4 shows a small portion of one organization's software-enabled ranking and scoring report. The report includes both quantitative financial indicators (e.g., NPV, internal rate of return) and qualitative measures (e.g., strategic new business growth, patient and physician satisfaction).

Through integrated evaluation, the organization's capital management council can link financial and capital plans to the organization's strategic plan and evaluate a potential capital portfolio to ensure it generates or saves enough cash for

Exhibit 9.4 Sample Report for Ranking and Scoring Capital Requests

Department	Description	Manager Rank	Executive Rank	Total Requested	NPV	Return Efficiency	First Year Positive Cash Flow	Internal Rate of Return	Payback	Average Score	Impact on Patient and/or Physician Satisfaction	Quality, Safety, & Compliance Effectiveness	Strategic & New Business Growth	Impact on Employee Work Experience
27200	MRI, New Equipment for Additional Capacity	1	5	1,950,000	(1,519,396)	-77.9%	NA	-14.8%	0.0	12.5	25	0	25	0
102002	General Construction, Dental Surgery Expansion	1	4	968,000	296,351	31.0%	2021	14.0%	6.8	81.3	100	75	75	75
102002	Other Respiratory Therapy, Hyperbaric Oxygen Chamber	3	2	1,010,800	894,928	89.0%	2019	24.0%	4.2	12.5	50	0	0	0
102002	Other Surgery, Stryker Targeting System	2	3	555,000	(844,190)	-152.0%	NA	0.0%	0.0	43.8	25	50	50	50
27640	General Renovation, OR Remodel	1	4	1,000,000	(1,000,000)	-100.0%	NA	0.0%	0.0	37.5	50	50	25	25
27550	EMG (Spine Neuro), Cyber Knife	1	1	5,855,000	24,122	0.0%	2023	10.0%	8.2	93.8	100	100	75	100
27540	General Construction, Sleep Lab Expansion	1	4	1,125,000	2,514,119	223.0%	2018	35.0%	3.2	87.5	100	75	75	100
27400	General Construction, New Cardiac Center	1	2	14,250,000	5,514,471	39.0%	2020	17.0%	5.0	68.8	100	50	75	50
27250	Linear Accelerator, Replacement of Existing	1	8	8,445,000	(20,759)	0.0%	2023	10.0%	8.3	25.0	25	25	25	25
27210	CT Scanner, Defensive Volume Initiative	16	58	1,350,000	(587,636)	-43.5%	2025	1.3%	9.5	12.5	25	25	0	0
26830	General Construction, Dialysis Center with Op Lease	1	57	1,500,000	(1,741,774)	-116.1%	NA	0.0%	0.0	18.8	25	25	25	0
26810	Other GI, Endoscopic Room	1	3	3,015,000	2,989,936	99.0%	2020	22.0%	5.7	25.0	25	25	25	25
26780	Other Cardiology, Cath Lab Expansion	1	3	6,100,000	5,670,773	93.0%	2019	22.0%	4.7	18.8	25	25	25	0
26750	Mammography Unit, Digital Mammo Unit	1	15	540,000	998,946	185.0%	2019	29.0%	4.2	50.0	50	25	75	50
26480	Master Facility Plan, New Cancer Center	2	2	11,125,000	1,323,327	11.9%	2026	13.2%	9.8	50.0	50	50	75	25
26440	General Construction, Third Floor NICU	1	1	1,876,000	253,820	14.0%	2020	12.0%	5.8	43.8	25	50	75	25
21010	Acquisition, SW MOB Acquisition	1	1	1,951,000	464,225	24.0%	2021	13.0%	6.9	62.5	75	50	75	50
19150	General Software, ICU Software	1	1	1,600,000	(4,540,127)	-284.0%	NA	0.0%	0.0	31.3	50	25	25	25

Source: Kaufman, Hall & Associates, LLC. Used with permission.

future investment. Using technology to support this process helps to ensure that the allocation of capital is effective; efficient; and based on optimal, transparent decision making.

Monitoring of Capital Spending

To track and report on capital spending, organizations should leverage the same database and software tools and capabilities discussed above. Having timely access to reports that highlight actual and committed project spending to date against approved capital helps leaders monitor a project's progress and ensure that funds are tracking as expected. In addition, the increased transparency and accountability generated by this enhanced data availability provide an effective basis for process enforcement and continuous improvement.

Monitoring of actual capital spending can be supported by transaction-level financial reporting. Where appropriate, project sponsors should include commentary to highlight project milestones that have been achieved. By increasing the granularity of monitoring and reporting, management can significantly improve its ability to hold project sponsors accountable for project results and to develop mitigation strategies, if necessary.

The shift from resource-intensive, manual capital planning and tracking to a more automated process has a variety of other benefits, including

- ensuring that the right stakeholders are engaged in the review and decision-making processes;
- increasing transparency around the portfolio of approved capital projects and ensuring that all required costs have been considered;
- increasing collaboration among departments involved in project review, which enhances the accuracy of cost and scheduling estimates; and
- ensuring that actual and committed spending stay within approved spending limits by consistently identifying and including comprehensive project costs.

Ultimately, technology-enhanced capital tracking provides controls and visibility that enable an organization to effectively monitor the release of actual funds against approved project budgets and more fully quantify the amount of approved, carryforward capital and its impact on future capital availability. In this way, the organization can ensure that its capital is invested as planned and continues to be consistent with the organization's strategic and financial plans.

Exhibit 9.5 describes how one organization implemented and uses best-practice software tools.

Avera Health implemented new capital allocation and management software tools systemwide in 2013. Uniform software has provided numerous benefits, such as a standardized set of analytics for data collection and a common format for conducting evaluations and communicating results to the capital committee. It also has allowed finance executives to standardize how different types of projects are categorized and classified systemwide.

The software's automated process for reviewing proposed projects has ensured that similar information is provided for each proposed investment and with a sufficient level of detail to enable informed decision making. The tools also support consistent use of objective financial and qualitative measures with which to evaluate projects.

These uniform processes have brought multiple benefits to Avera Health. Leaders throughout the system can clearly see where the organization's capital is being invested. As a result, they can better manage and monitor approved investments and can drive initiatives that enhance individual regions and the system as a whole.

Strong support from senior administration and broad representation on the work group both were critical to the initiative's success. "It was important to have key stakeholders intimately involved in developing the process," says Mike Olson, Avera's vice president of financial planning. "It wasn't forced on them; they had real buy-in as to what the process was going to look and feel like."

Developing a process that is somewhat fluid was critical to allow improvements to be made and automation to be enhanced over time as the organization evolves. For example, Avera redesigned its rating scale for proposed projects in the second year of implementation, after its initial scale introduced too much variability. Under the current system, stakeholders rank projects on a simple three-point scale.

Source: Avera Health. Used with permission.

THE ROLE OF TRANSPARENT COMMUNICATION

Comprehensively and transparently communicating all aspects of the capital allocation and management process—including process steps, process methodologies, basic principles of corporate finance, project-based analysis, and the process calendar—is essential to success. The capital allocation and management process's potential impact on an organization's decision-making processes demands extensive communication among all those involved in the process, especially in the first few years of process implementation. For organization-wide knowledge and transparency, communication routes must be broad, deep, and multidirectional, encompassing the board of directors, senior management, department directors, and clinicians.

Although different organizations use different communication strategies, three basic types of communication are required for successful process implementation:

1. *Up-front communication*: This type of communication should fully describe the planned capital allocation and management process, including its objectives, timing, informational requirements, and approval structure. A description of all associated decision support tools should be provided with detailed education and instructions for their use.

2. *Ongoing communication*: As the capital allocation and management process unfolds, an organization should maintain a continuous stream of communication throughout all levels of the business. Ongoing communication helps to ensure that process steps are transparent, support tools are used properly, project delays are avoided where possible, the technical approach is consistent, and process or technical errors are corrected in a timely manner.

3. *Feedback*: As opportunities for process improvements are identified, an organization should have a structured means for noting them and providing updated, corrected information organization-wide. These communications should be funneled through a single source to ensure that information is disseminated consistently throughout the organization.

To implement the capital allocation and management process, an organization must carefully develop and execute an ongoing communication plan. The plan should describe how analyses will be evaluated, by whom, and with which criteria. Armed with full information, managers and staff can make enhanced, informed decisions regarding development of valid projects and be assured that allocation decisions will further the organization's objectives.

Effective supporting materials are vital as an ongoing reference. Written materials that describe the capital allocation and management process and how staff members can participate in it can be posted on the organization's intranet to support implementation and provide basic information on corporate finance principles. These materials should be aimed at middle and senior management and can be as basic as needed to encourage participation in the process. One organization recorded an educational presentation so that each new staff member could view the video as part of the orientation process. The video not only helps the organization educate new staff members, but also establishes the organizational importance of the capital allocation and management process.

Decentralizing the capital allocation and management process through education and communication also increases its efficiency and effectiveness. An organization can appoint champions in each unit or department who, armed with an understanding of the importance of the process and how it works, will provide support for process implementation and act as ongoing resources in individual units.

Exhibit 9.6 describes one organization's education and communication efforts, as well as its results.

THE ROLE OF A DISCIPLINED IMPLEMENTATION PLAN AND TIME FRAME

Complete implementation of a smoothly running best-practice capital allocation and management process is likely to take two or three years. During the first year, an organization should seek manager buy-in to the process as a step in the right direction. Buy-in involves managers adopting analytical tools and adhering to the process schedule. The first-year goals are to boost the organization's financial knowledge and to establish capital allocation and management as a standard component of the organization's decision-making process.

During the second year, as managers continue to learn about and work within the capital allocation and management process, the objective is to ensure that they apply the concepts and approaches to all areas of decision making.

By the third year, the process should evolve to become an integral part of managers' annual efforts. At this stage, managers automatically eliminate bad projects from the process and understand the critical link between strategic planning and financial planning.

To evaluate implementation progress, leaders should ask the following questions:

- Has the number of projects submitted "through the back door" declined or been eliminated?
- Are the requirements for project analysis effectively decreasing the number of politically based projects?
- Has the quality of project analysis improved since standardized project review requirements were established?
- Has the general caliber of submitted projects improved?
- Are the projects submitted more consistent with organizational strategy and more focused on market growth and overall return than before the process was implemented?

Exhibit 9.6 Continuous Education and Communication at UAB Health System

The University of Alabama at Birmingham (UAB) Health System, an academic healthcare system in Birmingham, Alabama, implemented a best-practice capital allocation and management process supported by high-quality tools in 2011.

According to Mary Beth Briscoe, CPA, MBA, FHFMA, FACHE, the chief financial officer of the system's flagship University of Alabama Hospital (University Hospital) and of the clinical operations of UAB Medicine, early efforts included extensive communications to get all relevant stakeholders involved and educated. "Given the nuances and complexities of the capital structure within a healthcare organization, especially an academic organization, you cannot adopt a cookie-cutter approach," says Briscoe. "To realize an effective organization-wide process, it must be iterative and adaptable to stakeholder needs and concerns. Understanding that there's only one 'pot of dollars' promotes communication and collaboration."

Messaging and communication at UAB Health System centered on the need for a redesigned process, explaining why that process would require more structure and how it would be refined to reflect the culture and the strategies of the organization. "We have worked to ensure our process is adaptable to an ever-changing stakeholder group," notes Briscoe. The involvement of many different stakeholders, including physicians in subcommittee work groups and at the capital oversight committee level, provides an opportunity for everyone to be fully aware of the organization's needs and challenges. "A well-defined mission and vision has helped our organization promote collaborative communication across clinical and nonclinical settings. When you have clear direction, decisions impacting capital investments become more manageable," says Briscoe.

Organization-wide communication addresses not only what the process is and how it is accomplished but also what projects were approved through the process and, just as important, what projects were not approved. "Our inability to fund a project does not imply it is without merit and unimportant to our overall mission and vision. Quite the opposite. As we communicate funded projects and their individual importance, we also note the significance of nonfunded projects and a willingness to reevaluate each in the future or in the event additional funds become available," says Briscoe.

Clarity and transparency are critical, Briscoe adds. With knowledge about a major infrastructure need, such as HVAC replacement or an electrical system improvement, a program director better understands why the department's request for a new piece of technology could not be approved that year. As understanding increases, the capital allocation process becomes a call to action. "If the capital process works as intended, our stakeholders understand that the relationship between revenues and expenses directly impacts our ability to effectively respond to the organization's operational and strategic capital needs in a manner supporting our overall vision to be the preferred academic medical center of the twenty-first century," concludes Briscoe.

Source: University of Alabama at Birmingham Health System. Used with permission.

If the answer to any or all of these questions is yes, the organization has made significant progress toward successfully implementing corporate finance–based capital allocation and management.

Exhibit 9.7 describes typical barriers to the successful rollout of a best-practice capital management process and strategies to overcome them.

As described throughout this book, the goal of a best-practice capital allocation and management process is to deploy the organization's capital in a way that best supports its overall strategy and generates additional capital capacity for future investment. An organization that aims only to survive may not actually survive, and it certainly will not achieve the levels of competitive performance needed to thrive. Every small step taken toward its investment goals helps the organization improve its competitive financial position and enables it to more effectively pursue its key strategies.

The capital allocation and management process must be designed to evolve. An organization should review the process annually to assess its progress toward meeting specified goals. To do this, the organization must look at what works and why, what does not work and why, what needs to be added, and which components are unnecessary and can be eliminated.

Process review should be a formal component of the process structure and should occur at approximately the same time each year. An organization must be willing and able to adjust the process to meet its evolving internal and external needs. For example, an organization might need to adjust the schedule, analytical components, and definitions of threshold and nonthreshold capital. Individuals participating in the process at both the leadership and department levels should be empowered to suggest necessary changes to enhance the process.

Ultimately, the most important factor for a successful capital allocation and management process is patience. As mentioned earlier, two or three years likely will pass before the process runs as designed. Ingrained organizational behavior cannot be altered quickly—especially behavior that is integral to an organization's operations and politics. In many organizations, capital-related decisions are highly politicized, providing benefits to key constituencies in the organization. Implementing a corporate finance–based capital allocation and management process in these organizations will likely represent a significant change. Making that change and achieving optimal results will take time.

IMPLEMENTATION CONSIDERATIONS

Organizations must navigate a changing business model. To do this, they must adopt effective decision-making processes.

Exhibit 9.7 Barriers to a Successful Rollout of Best-Practice Capital Allocation and Management and Strategies to Overcome Them

Avoidance

"The process involves too much work," many staff members complain. This barrier results from a lack of awareness of the magnitude of the decisions being made and the implications of inappropriate decisions. Overcoming this objection is accomplished through transparency—by providing information about the variety and significance of the investments being evaluated. If the projects are not worth the up-front analysis, why would they be worth the investment?

Misperception

"My project is different and shouldn't have to go through the usual capital management process," some people grumble. This barrier is exacerbated in an environment in which decision making does not employ an analytical, corporate finance–based approach. Use of the common language of NPV, described in chapter 6, and other corporate finance tools can address this challenge. The objective quantification of financial return and the application of portfolio-based decision making ensures that each project is evaluated on an equal footing.

Misunderstanding

"This is a defensive project—its benefits cannot be quantified," some sponsors protest. This barrier reflects the classic politics that often characterize capital decision making. By claiming the project's unique ability to defend the organization, the project champion moves the decision from an analytical framework to a political and emotional one. This is especially true of projects with little or no potential return. To overcome this barrier, leaders can ask project owners to quantify those aspects of the project that can be quantified, specifically including the cost of not investing in it.

Subversion

"I will just go to the CEO; the CEO always approves what I want," some staff say to themselves. This barrier can be overcome simply by the CEO's explicit endorsement and adoption of the formal capital allocation and management process. This endorsement forces decisions out of the hallway or private office and into a public conference room.

Source: Kaufman, Hall & Associates, LLC. Used with permission.

Capital allocation and management is not a matter of convenience, but a matter of necessity. Organizational culture must focus on integrated decision making that encompasses strategic and financial planning, capital allocation and management, and budgeting and performance reporting.

Capital allocation and management decisions are larger than any single individual, affecting every department and every function in an organization. The processes described in this book require the direct input and participation of individuals with many diverse skill sets in many different organizational roles.

There is no better time than now to start this journey, but organizations must establish reasonable and realistic goals for their transformation. The design process will identify characteristics and components of an ideal state. The plan to fully implement that ideal state, however, may require a multiple-cycle or multiple-year horizon.

Closing Comments

AN EFFECTIVE CAPITAL allocation and management process is organized around the concepts described in this book—articulated objectives and principles; defined, standardized methodologies; clear governance and accountability; a known calendar; effective implementation; and ongoing education and communication.

Implementing a rigorous, corporate finance–based capital management and allocation process represents a significant organizational change for most healthcare organizations—a change that is often unwelcome. Managers or executives who are accustomed to making independent capital decisions may resist the new process, and its iterative nature may lead to frustration.

The benefits of a best-practice process, however, are well worth the effort of meeting these challenges. The discipline, rigor, and analytic standards of a best-practice capital management process help all constituents recognize the importance of proactively managing capital spending. The collaborative and transparent nature of the process gives the organization a strategic focus and ensures organization-wide consistency in spending.

A best-practice process fully integrates strategic planning with financial and capital planning. Capital can be approved based on the alignment of proposed investments with strategic goals and within established financial and risk parameters; capital can be denied based on concrete strategic and financial reasons rather than on political positioning.

An improved process not only identifies projects most likely to bring strategic and financial success to an organization but also keeps bad ideas off the table. The result is fewer "disastrous initiatives" in the long term and an improved bottom line.

Will organizations continue to maintain good capital allocation and management processes when they have good bottom lines, or will they become undisciplined? Will profitability be sustainable? In almost all healthcare organizations, capital appetites routinely exceed capital constraints. This fact creates a continued need for a disciplined best-practice capital allocation and management process, even in the best and worst of times. Choices will always need to be made. Political influence will always need to be countered by the discipline provided by corporate finance–based decision making.

Circling back to this book's opening words, in an environment of scarce resources, increasing competition, and significant requirements for capital investment, healthcare executives must allocate available capital to initiatives that will best meet the strategic objectives of their organization while enhancing its financial performance. The best-practice capital allocation and management process described in this book offers an effective approach to making the decisions that will ensure their organization's competitive performance, both strategically and financially. Implement the approach. Advance the discipline.

About the Author

Jason H. Sussman is a managing director at Kaufman, Hall & Associates, LLC, where he directs capital planning and allocation advisory services in the firm's strategic and financial planning practice. His experience includes all aspects of financial planning and provision of financial advisory services to hospitals, healthcare systems, and physician groups nationwide. His areas of expertise include strategic financial planning, capital allocation and management, mergers and acquisitions, financing transactions, and management software.

Prior to joining Kaufman, Hall & Associates, LLC, in 1990, Mr. Sussman directed the Chicago capital finance group of a national accounting firm's healthcare consulting practice. Previously, he was the special assistant to the president at Michael Reese Hospital and Medical Center in Chicago, responsible for the institution's certificate-of-need and capital budgeting processes.

In addition to the first edition of this book, *The Healthcare Executive's Guide to Allocating Capital* (Chicago: Health Administration Press, 2007), Mr. Sussman has authored articles for a variety of industry periodicals, including *Healthcare Financial Management* magazine, and was a contributing author to *Best-Practice Financial Management: Six Key Concepts for Healthcare Leaders* (Chicago: Health Administration Press, 2006) and *The Financially Competitive Healthcare Organization* (Chicago: Probus Publishing, 1994). He has presented programs at seminars sponsored by the American College of Healthcare Executives (ACHE), the American Hospital Association, the Healthcare Financial Management Association (HFMA), the National Association of Children's Hospitals and Related Institutions, and several state hospital associations.

Mr. Sussman holds a master of business administration degree in finance and accounting, with a specialization in healthcare management, from Northwestern University's Kellogg Graduate School of Management in Evanston, Illinois, and a bachelor of arts degree from the Johns Hopkins University in Baltimore, Maryland. He is a certified public accountant in Illinois and a member of ACHE and HFMA.